AF181896

Inflammatory Heart Diseases

Edited by Wilbert S. Aronow and Takashi Murashita

Published in London, United Kingdom

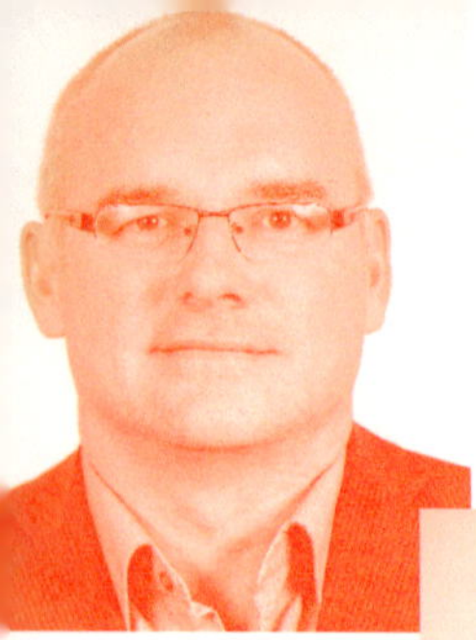
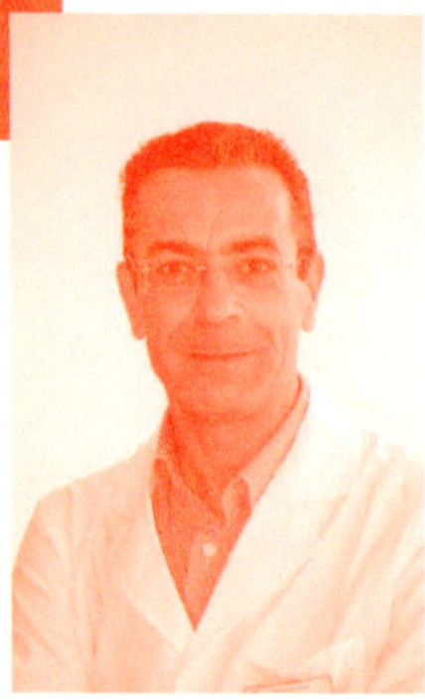
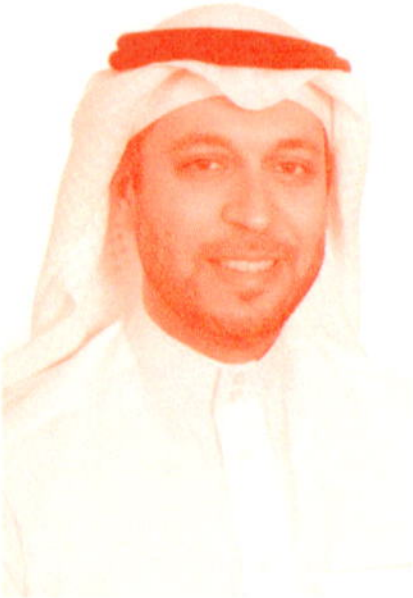
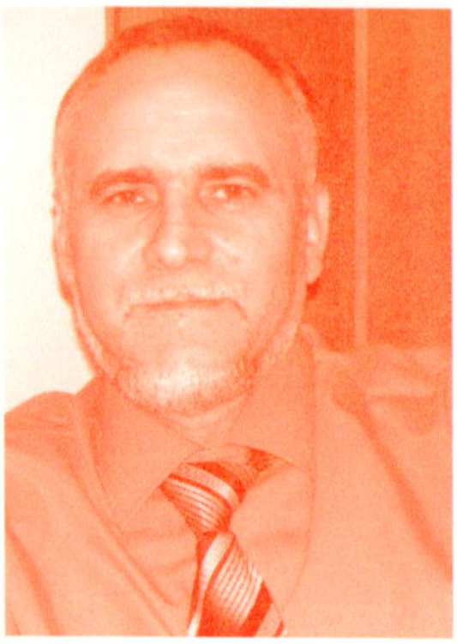
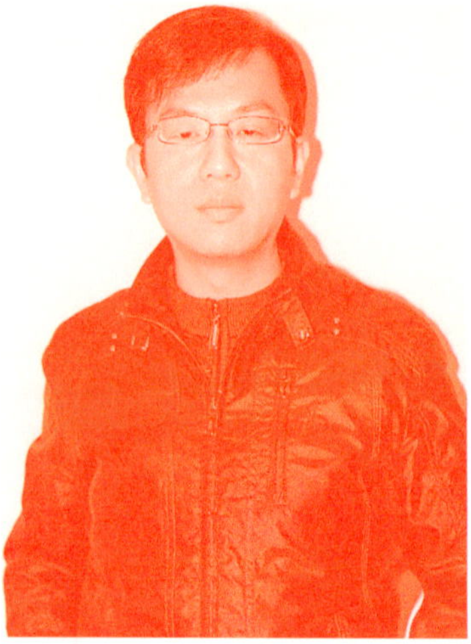
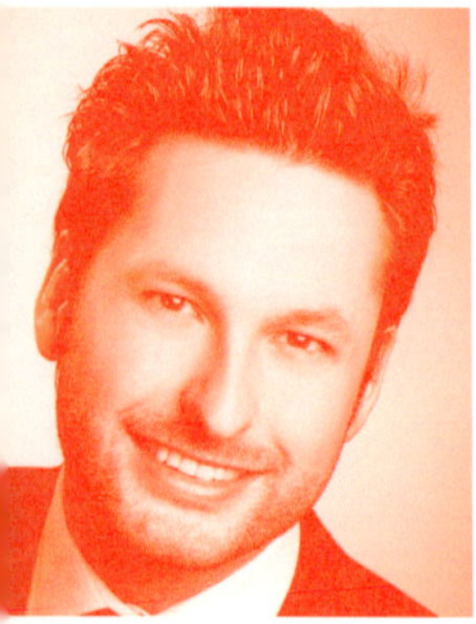
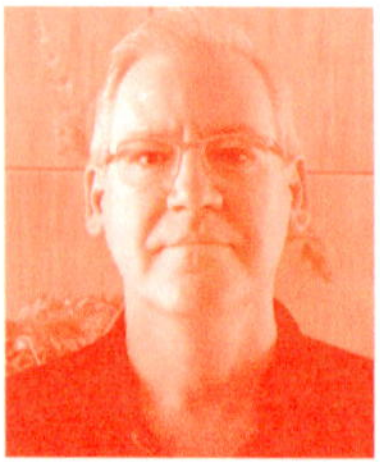

IntechOpen

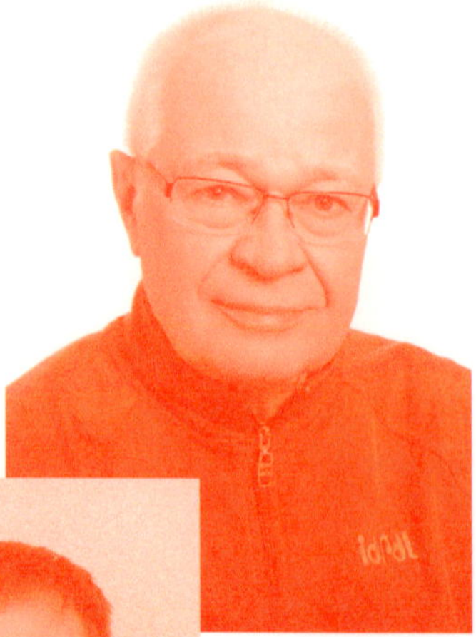
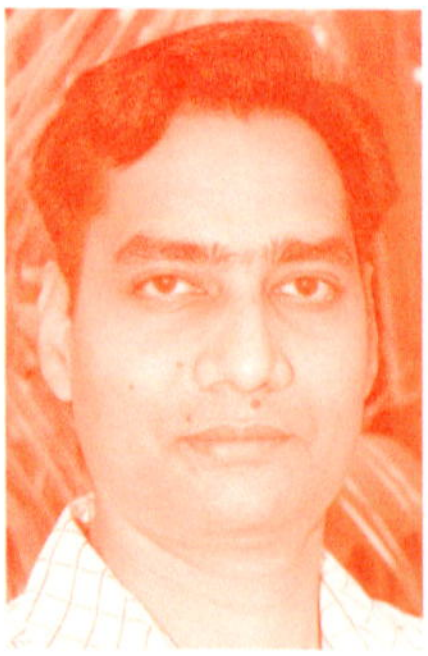
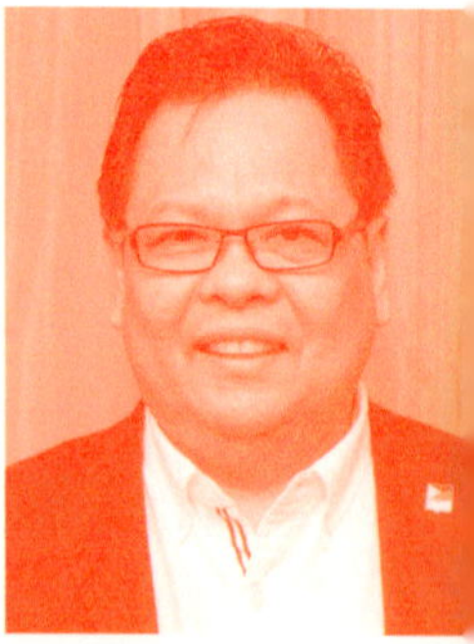
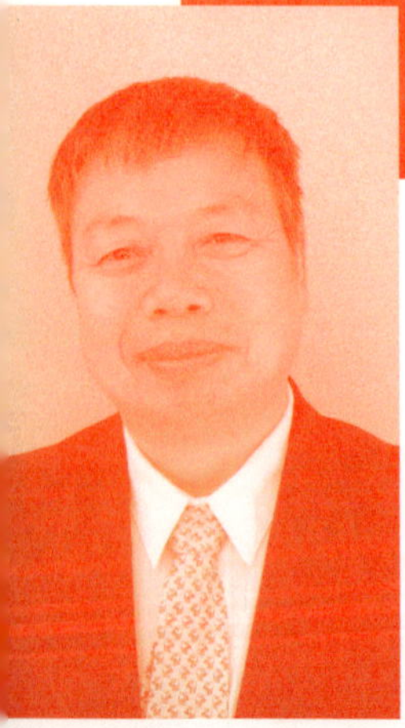
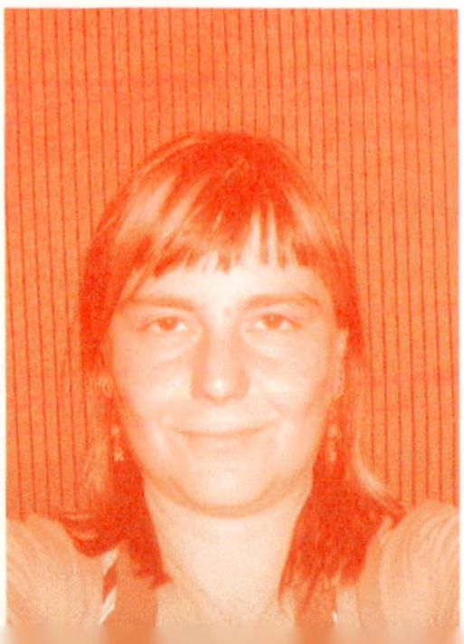
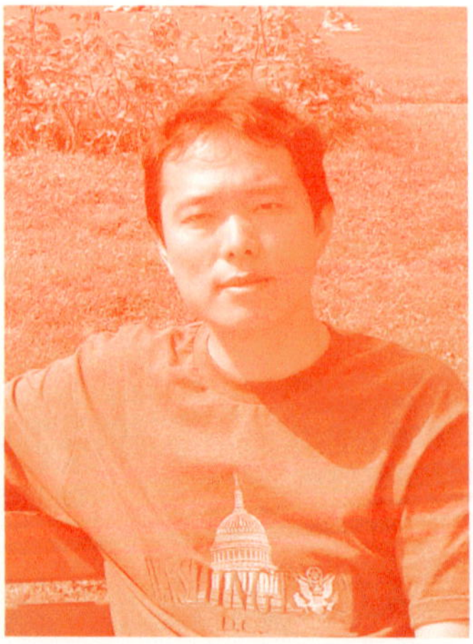

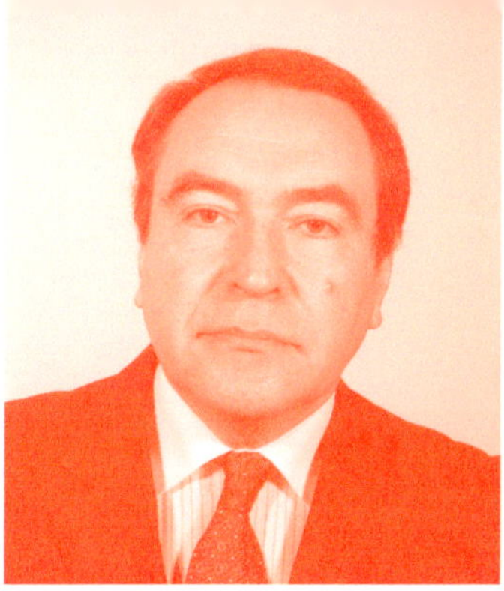
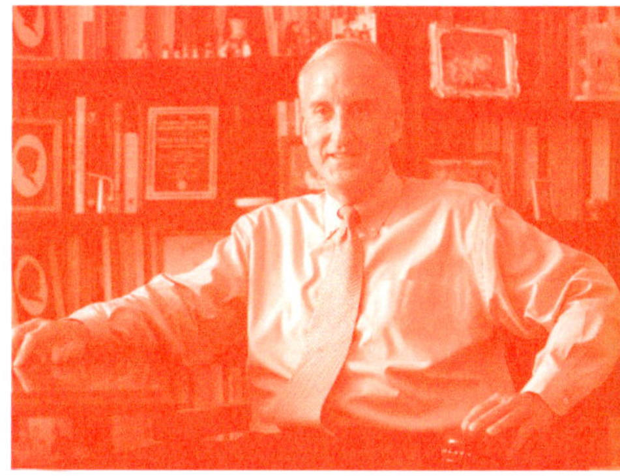
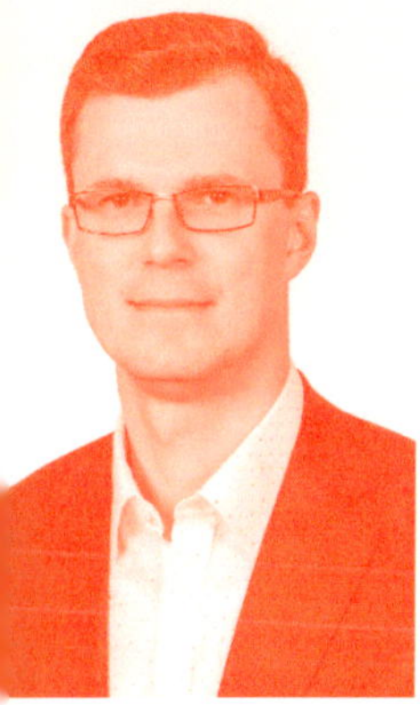
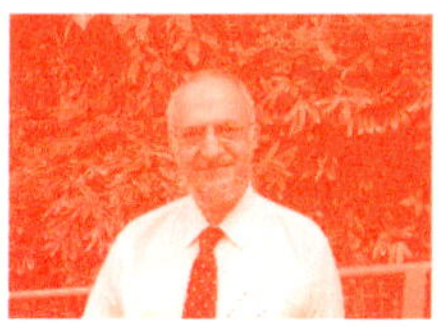
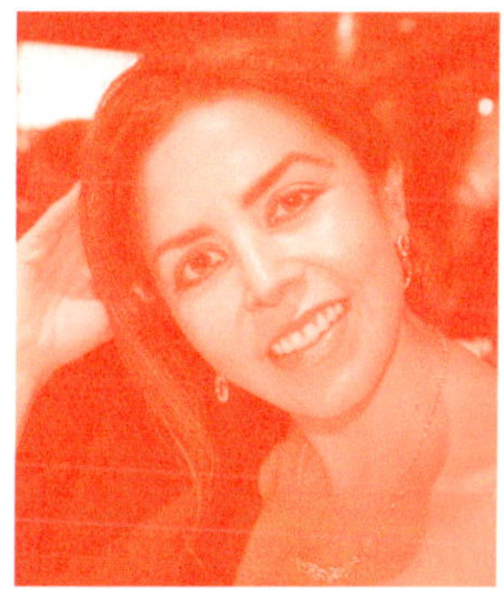

Supporting open minds since 2005

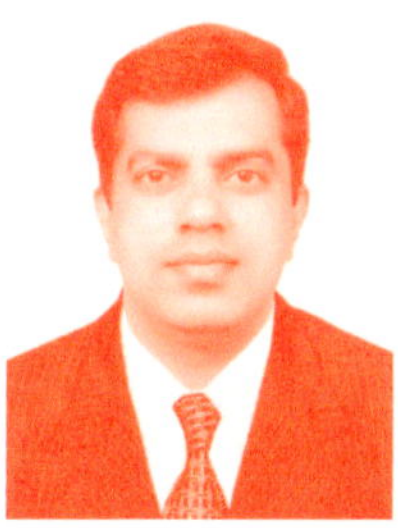
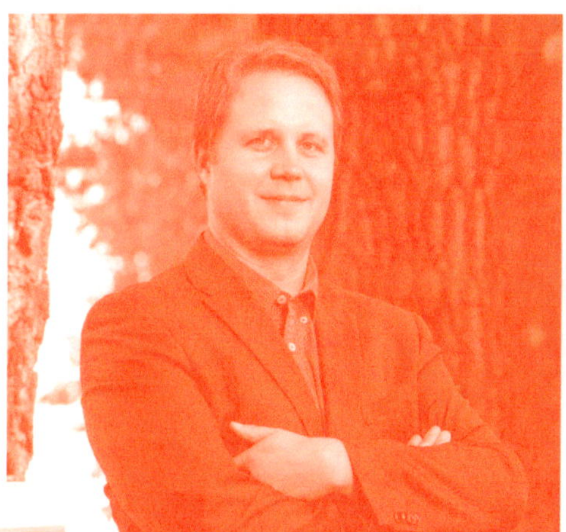
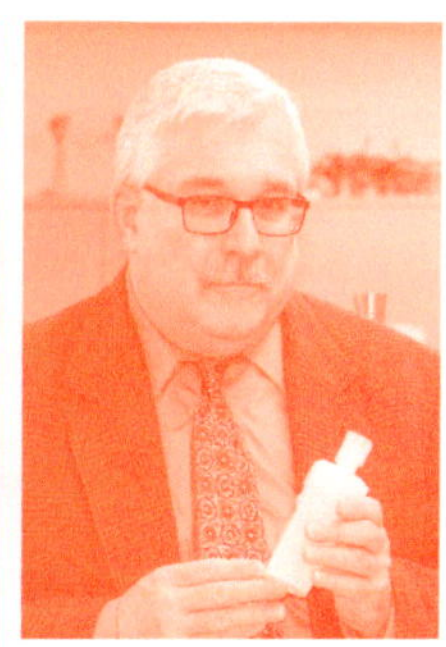
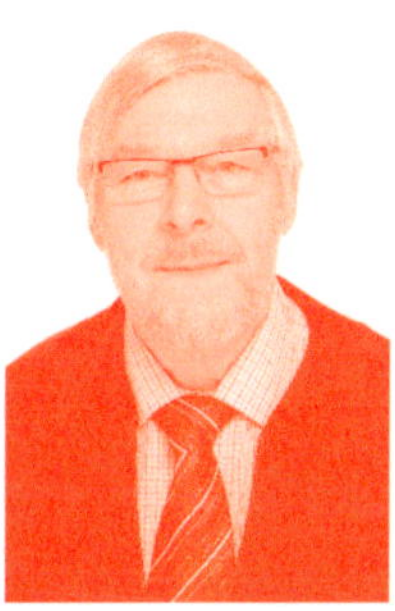
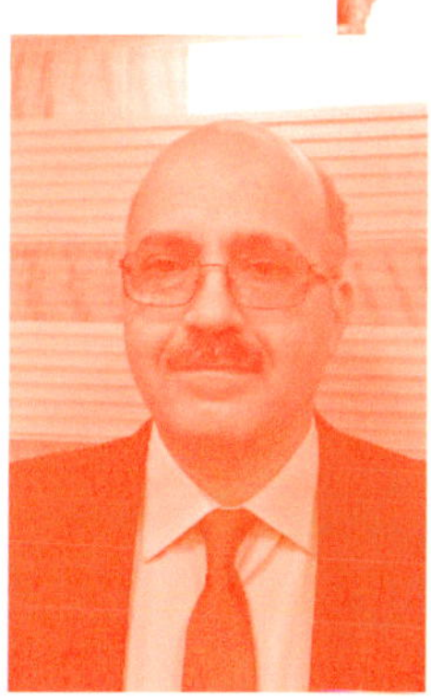
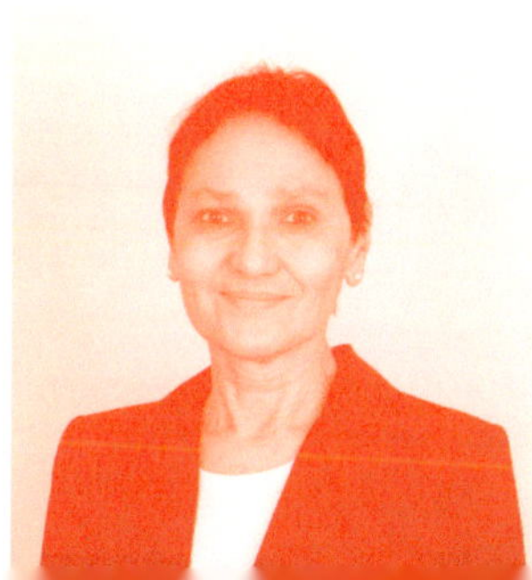
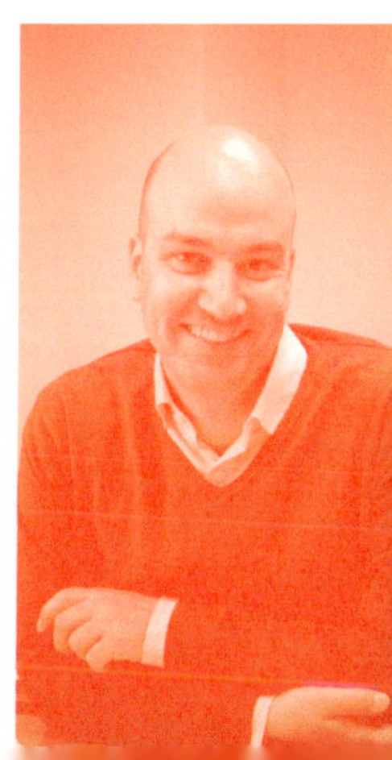

Inflammatory Heart Diseases
http://dx.doi.org/10.5772/intechopen.77708
Edited by Wilbert S. Aronow and Takashi Murashita

Contributors
Herve Yangni-Angate, Ing Xiang Soo, Michelle Correia, Nissar Shaikh, Jose Picco, Yousif Mohamed Y. Mohamed Yousif Abdallah, Nouf Abuhadi, Takashi Murashita, Sushama Bhosale, Sharon Tai, Wilbert S. Aronow, Kartik Dhaduk, Ammar Athar, Jaipaul Singh, Frank Christopher Howarth, Manal M. A. Smail, Abla M Ismail

© The Editor(s) and the Author(s) 2019
The rights of the editor(s) and the author(s) have been asserted in accordance with the Copyright, Designs and Patents Act 1988. All rights to the book as a whole are reserved by INTECHOPEN LIMITED. The book as a whole (compilation) cannot be reproduced, distributed or used for commercial or non-commercial purposes without INTECHOPEN LIMITED's written permission. Enquiries concerning the use of the book should be directed to INTECHOPEN LIMITED rights and permissions department (permissions@intechopen.com).
Violations are liable to prosecution under the governing Copyright Law.

Individual chapters of this publication are distributed under the terms of the Creative Commons Attribution 3.0 Unported License which permits commercial use, distribution and reproduction of the individual chapters, provided the original author(s) and source publication are appropriately acknowledged. If so indicated, certain images may not be included under the Creative Commons license. In such cases users will need to obtain permission from the license holder to reproduce the material. More details and guidelines concerning content reuse and adaptation can be found at http://www.intechopen.com/copyright-policy.html.

Notice
Statements and opinions expressed in the chapters are these of the individual contributors and not necessarily those of the editors or publisher. No responsibility is accepted for the accuracy of information contained in the published chapters. The publisher assumes no responsibility for any damage or injury to persons or property arising out of the use of any materials, instructions, methods or ideas contained in the book.

First published in London, United Kingdom, 2019 by IntechOpen
IntechOpen is the global imprint of INTECHOPEN LIMITED, registered in England and Wales, registration number: 11086078, 7th floor, 10 Lower Thames Street, London, EC3R 6AF, United Kingdom
Printed in Croatia

British Library Cataloguing-in-Publication Data
A catalogue record for this book is available from the British Library

Additional hard and PDF copies can be obtained from orders@intechopen.com

Inflammatory Heart Diseases
Edited by Wilbert S. Aronow and Takashi Murashita
p. cm.
Print ISBN 978-1-78985-275-2
Online ISBN 978-1-78985-276-9
eBook (PDF) ISBN 978-1-83968-238-4

For EU product safety concerns:
IN TECH d.o.o., Prolaz Marije Krucifikse Kozulić 3, 51000 Rijeka, Croatia, info@intechopen.com or visit our website at intechopen.com.

We are IntechOpen, the world's leading publisher of Open Access books

Built by scientists, for scientists

4,500+
Open access books available

118,000+
International authors and editors

130M+
Downloads

151
Countries delivered to

Our authors are among the
Top 1%
most cited scientists

12.2%
Contributors from top 500 universities

CLARIVATE ANALYTICS
BOOK CITATION INDEX
INDEXED

WEB OF SCIENCE™

Selection of our books indexed in the Book Citation Index
in Web of Science™ Core Collection (BKCI)

Interested in publishing with us?
Contact book.department@intechopen.com

Numbers displayed above are based on latest data collected.
For more information visit www.intechopen.com

Meet the editors

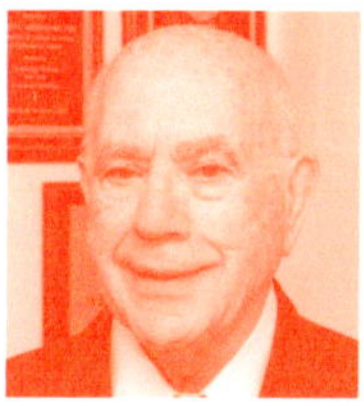

Wilbert S. Aronow, MD, is Professor of Medicine and Director of Cardiology Research at Westchester Medical Center and New York Medical College Valhalla, NY, USA. He received his MD from Harvard Medical School. He has edited 17 books and is author or co-author of 1727 papers or book chapters, 610 commentaries, 47 Letters to the Editor, and 1137 abstracts. He has also presented or co-presented 1510 talks at meetings. He is a Fellow of the American College of Cardiology (ACC), the America Heart Association (AHA), the American College of Physicians (ACP), the American College of Clinical Pharmacy (ACCP), the American Society for Preventive Cardiology (ASPC), the AGS (Founding Fellow of Western Section) , and the GSA. He has been an editorial board member for 179 medical journals. He has been a member of four national guidelines committees including the 2010 AMDA guidelines for heart failure, the 2011 ACC/AHA expert consensus document on hypertension in the elderly, the 2015 AHA/ACC/ASH scientific statement on treatment of hypertension in patients with coronary artery disease, and the 2017 ACC/AHA guidelines for the management of patients with hypertension.

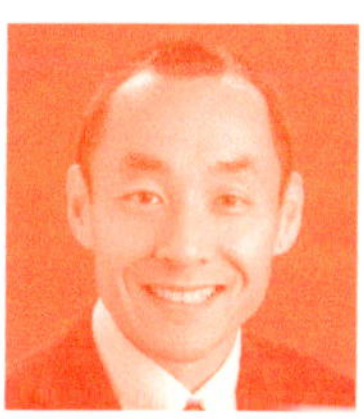

Takashi Murashita, MD, is an assistant professor in the Department of Surgery at the University of Missouri, Columbia, MO, USA. Dr. Murashita received his MD from Kyoto University Medical School, Japan. His main interest is cardiac surgery, and he is a member of the Society of Thoracic Surgery, Eastern Cardiothoracic Surgical Society, and Asian Society for Cardiovascular and Thoracic Surgery. He has published 52 papers in peer-reviewed journals and nine book chapters in open access journals. He has been an editorial board member for two medical journals and an ad-hoc manuscript reviewer for fifteen medical journals.

Contents

Preface

Inflammatory Heart Diseases, edited by Drs. Aronow and Murashita, presents comprehensive information on pericardial diseases, cardiomyopathies, and atherosclerotic cardiovascular diseases.

In the first section, chapters cover advanced concepts in pericardial disease, pericardial disease in the elderly, tuberculous pericarditis, surgical treatment of chronic constrictive pericarditis, surgery for chronic pericardial effusion, and anesthesia for patients with pericardial disease.

In the second section, chapters discuss inflammation and diabetic cardiomyopathy, peripartum cardiomyopathies, and medical imaging in myocarditis.

In the third section, chapters examine atherosclerosis of extracranial carotid vessels and serum homocysteine, and the role of lifestyle in the development of coronary heart disease.

I would like to thank all of the contributors for their outstanding work. I would also like to acknowledge the excellent editing of Professor Murashita and the excellent assistance of Sara Bacvarova, Author Service Manager at IntechOpen.

Wilbert S. Aronow, MD, FACC, FAHA
Professor of Medicine and Director of Cardiology Research,
Westchester Medical Center and New York Medical College

Section 1

Pericarditis

Chapter 1

Prologue: Introduction to Advanced Concepts in Pericardial Disease

Takashi Murashita

1. Introduction

Pericardial diseases are common in clinical practice and include a variety of pathologies such as pericarditis (acute, subacute, chronic, and recurrent), pericardial effusion, cardiac tamponade, constrictive pericarditis, and pericardial masses [1, 2]. The etiology of pericardial diseases is classified into infectious, autoimmune, post-myocardial infarction, and autoreactive causes. When etiology is not apparent, it is classified as idiopathic. Multimodality imaging is an essential approach for a modern and comprehensive diagnostic evaluation [3]. The goal of this text is to highlight the current concepts in the clinical characteristics, presentation, diagnosis, and the treatment for pericardial diseases.

2. Pericarditis

2.1 Acute pericarditis

Acute pericarditis can be diagnosed with at least two of the four following criteria: (1) pericarditic chest pain, (2) pericardial rubs, (3) new widespread ST elevation or PR depression on electrocardiogram, and (4) pericardial effusion (new or worsening). The additional supporting findings include (1) elevation of inflammation markers (C-reactive protein, erythrocyte sedimentation rate, and white blood cell count) and (2) evidence of pericardial inflammation shown by computed tomography or magnetic resonance imaging.

In developing countries, tuberculosis is the leading cause of pericarditis, and it is often associated with HIV infection. In developed countries, more than 80% of the cases are idiopathic, and the cause is often presumed as viral infection [2].

In terms of diagnosis of suspected acute pericarditis, electrocardiogram, transthoracic echocardiogram, chest X-ray, and assessment of inflammation markers and myocardial injury are recommended as a class I indication [1].

Predictors of poor prognosis for acute pericarditis include (1) fever >38°C, (2) subacute onset, (3) large pericardial effusion, (4) cardiac tamponade, and (5) lack of response to aspirin or nonsteroidal anti-inflammatory drugs (NSAIDs) after at least 1 week of therapy. If the patients are categorized in high risk (at least one risk factor of above), hospital admission is recommended. Outpatient management is recommended for low-risk patients.

Regarding treatment, aspirin or NSAIDs are recommended as first-line therapy with gastroprotection. Colchicine is also recommended as first-line therapy as an

IntechOpen

adjunct to aspirin/NSAID therapy (**Table 1**). Evaluation of response to anti-inflammatory therapy is recommended after 1 week. Low-dose corticosteroids can be considered in cases of contraindication/failure of aspirin/NSAIDs and colchicine, when an infectious cause is excluded or when there is a specific indication such as an autoimmune disease.

2.2 Recurrent pericarditis

Recurrent pericarditis is the most common complication of acute pericarditis, and it happens in 30% of patients with a first attack of acute pericarditis. Recurrent pericarditis is defined with a symptom-free interval of 4–6 weeks or longer after the first episode of acute pericarditis.

Diagnosis is established by C-reactive protein, computed tomography, and/or cardiac magnetic resonance imaging showing pericardial inflammation.

Commonly prescribed anti-inflammatory therapies for recurrent pericarditis are aspirin, ibuprofen, indomethacin, and colchicine (**Table 2**). Colchicine is recommended for at least 6 months. In cases of incomplete response to aspirin/NSAIDs and colchicine, corticosteroids may be used. However, severe side effects of corticosteroids were reported in about 25% of patients with high oral dose of corticosteroids. In order to avoid systemic side effects of corticosteroids, the intrapericardial route has been proposed [4, 5]; however, this technique requires further investigation. Drugs such as immunoglobulin, anakinra, or azathioprine are considered as third-line therapy in cases of non-response to aspirin/NSAIDS, colchicine, or

Drug	Usual dosing	Therapy duration	Tapering
Aspirin	750–1000 mg every 8 hours	1–2 weeks	Decrease doses by 250–500 mg every 1–2 weeks
Ibuprofen	600 mg every 8 hours	1–2 weeks	Decrease doses by 250–500 mg every 1–2 weeks
Colchicine	0.5 mg per day (<70 kg) 0.5 mg twice a day (≥70 kg)	3 months	Not mandatory

Table 1.
Commonly prescribed anti-inflammatory therapy for acute pericarditis.

Drug	Usual dosing	Therapy duration	Tapering
Aspirin	500–1000 mg every 6–8 hours	Weeks–months	Decrease doses by 250–500 mg every 1–2 weeks
Ibuprofen	600 mg every 8 hours	Weeks–months	Decrease doses by 200–400 mg every 1–2 weeks
Indomethacin	25–50 mg every 8 hours	Weeks–months	Decrease doses by 25 mg every 1–2 weeks
Colchicine	0.5 mg per day (<70 kg) 0.5 mg twice a day (≥70 kg)	At least 6 months	Not mandatory

Table 2.
Commonly prescribed anti-inflammatory therapy for recurrent pericarditis.

corticosteroids. As a last resort, pericardiectomy is considered after a thorough trail of unsuccessful medical therapy.

C-reactive protein dosage should be considered to guide the treatment duration and assess the response to therapy. After the normalization of C-reactive protein, a gradual tapering of therapies should be considered, tailored to symptoms, stopping a single class of drugs at a time.

2.3 Myopericarditis

Pericarditis which has concomitant myocardial involvement is referred to as myopericarditis. The classical presentation of myopericarditis is chest pain with other signs of pericarditis, in addition to the elevation of markers of myocardial damage. Viral infections are the most common cause in developed countries, whereas infectious causes such as tuberculosis are common in developing countries.

In cases of suspected myopericarditis, coronary angiography is recommended in order to rule out acute coronary syndrome. Cardiac magnetic resonance is also recommended for the confirmation of myocardial involvement. Hospitalization, rest, and avoidance of physical activity beyond normal sedentary activities are recommended in nonathletes and athletes with myopericarditis for a period of 6 months.

3. Pericardial effusion and cardiac tamponade

Pericardial effusion is classified according to onset as acute, subacute, and chronic when lasting >3 months. The pericardial effusion, which was caused by inflammation leading to increased production of pericardial fluid, is called exudate pericardial effusion. On the other hand, the accumulation of pericardial fluid caused by decrease reabsorption due to an increase in systemic venous pressure as a result of congestive heart failure or pulmonary hypertension is called transudate pericardial effusion.

As of diagnosis, transthoracic echocardiography is recommended (**Figure 1**), and it can assess the size of the pericardial effusion (mild, < 10 mm; moderate, 10–20 mm; or large, > 20 mm), distribution (circumferential or loculated), and hemodynamic effects.

Pericardial effusion is often associated with known or unknown medical conditions such as infections (viral, bacterial, and tuberculosis), cancer, connective

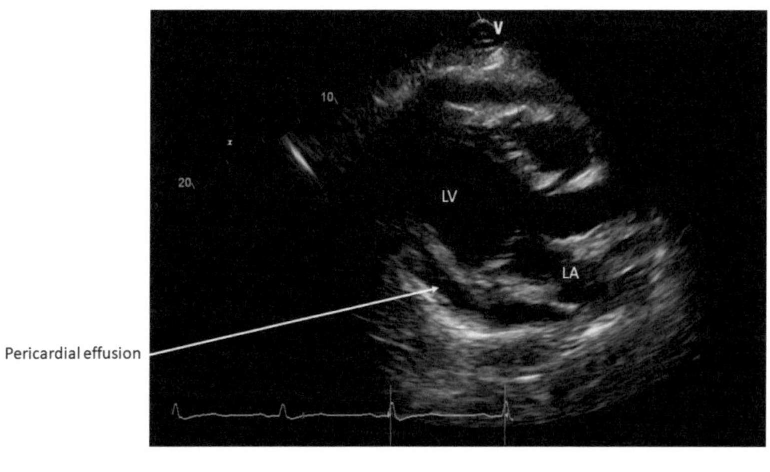

Figure 1.
The echocardiographic imaging for pericardial effusion. LA, left atrium; LV, left ventricle.

tissue diseases, trauma, and metabolic causes (e.g., hypothyroidism). In developed countries, over 50% of the etiology is idiopathic, whereas tuberculosis is the leading etiology in developing countries.

It is recommended that the therapy of pericardial effusion is targeted at the etiology. When pericardial effusion is associated with systemic inflammation, aspirin/NSAIDs/colchicine, and treatment of pericarditis are recommended. For cardiac tamponade, symptomatic moderate to large pericardial effusions not responsive to medical therapy, and suspicion of unknown bacterial or neoplastic etiology, pericardiocentesis or pericardial window is indicated.

The common causes of cardiac tamponade include pericarditis, tuberculosis, iatrogenesis (invasive procedure-related, post-cardiac surgery), trauma, and neoplasm/malignancy. The other causes include autoimmune diseases (systemic lupus erythematosus, rheumatoid arthritis, scleroderma), radiation, post-myocardial infarction, uremia, aortic dissection, bacterial infection, and pneumopericardium.

4. Constrictive pericarditis

Constrictive pericarditis is a result from inflammation and fibrosis of the pericardium leading to diastolic dysfunction and right heart failure. Generally speaking, constrictive pericarditis is irreversible, and once the diagnosis is made, surgical pericardiectomy is indicated in patients with symptoms of heart failure.

In Western countries, the etiology of constrictive pericarditis is mainly idiopathic, presumably unrecognized prior viral pericarditis. Previous cardiac surgery and prior mediastinal radiation therapy are becoming more popular. On the other hand, tuberculosis is a major cause of constrictive pericarditis in developing countries.

In constrictive pericarditis, Kussmaul sign and pericardial knock are common physical findings. Electrocardiogram may show low voltages, non-specific ST-T changes, or atrial fibrillation. Chest X-ray shows pericardial calcification in one-third of the cases.

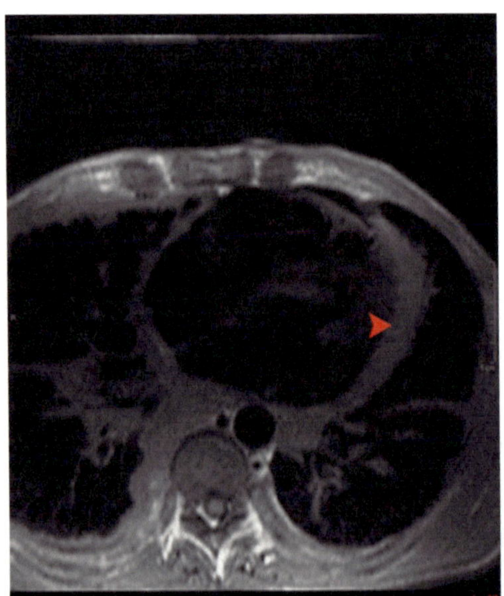

Figure 2.
Cardiac magnetic resonance imaging shows thickening of the pericardium (arrow).

Syndrome	Definition	Therapy
Transient constriction	Reversible pattern of constriction following spontaneous recovery or medical therapy	2–3 months of empiric anti-inflammatory drugs
Effusive-constrictive pericarditis	Failure of the right atrial pressure to fall by 50% or to a level below 10 mmHg after pericardiocentesis	Pericardiocentesis followed by medical therapy. Surgery for persistent cases
Chronic constriction	Persistent constriction after 3–6 months	Pericardiectomy, medical therapy for advanced cases or high risk of surgery, or mixed forms with myocardial involvement

Table 3.
Definition and therapy for constrictive pericarditis.

For the diagnosis of constrictive pericarditis, transthoracic echocardiography and chest X-ray with adequate technical characteristics are recommended in all patients with suspected constrictive pericarditis. Echocardiography may show septal bounce, pericardial thickening and calcifications, respiratory variation of the mitral peak E velocity of >25% and variation in the pulmonary venous peak D flow velocity of >20%, or color M-mode flow propagation velocity > 45 cm/s. Computed tomography and cardiac magnetic resonance imaging are indicated as second-level imaging techniques to assess calcifications, pericardial thickness (3–4 mm), degree, and extension of pericardial involvement (**Figure 2**). Cardiac catheterization may show "dip and plateau" sign, right ventricular diastolic and left ventricular diastolic pressures usually equal, and ventricular independence.

The definitions and therapy of the main constrictive pericarditis are listed in **Table 3**.

5. Surgical treatment for pericardial disease

5.1 Pericardial window

A pericardial window is the procedure to create a communication from the pericardial space to the pleural space. The purpose of this procedure is to allow a pericardial effusion (usually malignant) to drain from the pericardial space into the chest cavity to prevent a large accumulation of pericardial fluid and cardiac tamponade.

Subxiphoid pericardial window is done by either local or general anesthesia. A vertical incision about 4 cm is made over the xiphoid process and upper abdomen. The diaphragm is dissected away from the undersurface of the sternum and xiphoid, fat is removed from over the pericardium, and the pericardium is opened under direct vision. All fluid is aspirated, and loculations may be broken up gently with the sucker. As large a pericardial window as possible is made by excision of the pericardium. Pericardial tissue and fluid are sent for bacteriologic and histologic study.

Another way to do a pericardial window is via a left anterolateral approach. A small left anterolateral incision is made, and a simple pericardial window is created, usually of necessity anterior to the phrenic nerve. After evacuation of fluid, chest tubes are placed in the pleural space.

5.2 Pericardiectomy

Pericardiectomy is indicated in patients with symptomatic constrictive pericarditis, especially those patients requiring increasing doses of diuretics. It is also indicated in patients with effusive-constrictive pericarditis who do not respond to anti-inflammatory medications.

Pericardiectomy is typically done through median sternotomy, whereas it can be done via left anterolateral or bilateral thoracotomy. Complete pericardiectomy is defined as removal of the whole pericardium overlying the heart and proximal great vessels except for the pericardium posterior to the left atrium in the oblique sinus and variable amounts of pericardium adjacent to the phrenic nerves. Thus, the anterior pericardium (phrenic nerve to phrenic nerve), the diaphragmatic pericardium, and a portion of the pericardium posterior to the left phrenic nerve should be removed. Failure to remove the pericardium from the diaphragmatic surface may lead to late recurrence of constrictive physiology.

Although cardiopulmonary bypass and systemic heparinization may increase the risk of bleeding, decompression of the heart with extracorporeal circulation is useful and necessary in many patients because circulatory support facilitates dissection of the pericardium and allows wide manipulation of the ventricles. Further, with cardiopulmonary bypass, any injury to the myocardium is more easily repaired. Another advantage is that during cardiopulmonary bypass, the patient's total blood volume is drained into the cardiotomy reservoir, and after pericardiectomy, intravascular volume is adjusted to maintain adequate cardiac output and perfusion.

One of the largest number of pericardiectomy was reported from the Mayo Clinic [6]. They reviewed 1071 pericardiectomy operations for about 80 years. The etiology of constrictive pericarditis was idiopathic in 62%, post-cardiac surgery in 27%, and postradiation in 10% in the contemporary era. The 30-day mortality was 5.2% in the contemporary era and 13.5% in the historical era. The risk factors of overall mortality in the contemporary era were the New York Heart Association class III or IV, etiology of radiation or post-cardiac surgery, and the need for cardiopulmonary bypass.

6. Conclusions

Despite the recent advancement in diagnostic images and treatment options, there have been a limited number of randomized controlled studies in the field of pericardial disease. Therefore, contemporary management of pericardial disease is mainly performed empirically. Nowadays new diagnostic techniques have been available in the study of pericardial diseases.

Author details

Takashi Murashita
University of Missouri, Columbia, Missouri, USA

*Address all correspondence to: tmurashita@gmail.com

IntechOpen

© 2019 The Author(s). Licensee IntechOpen. This chapter is distributed under the terms of the Creative Commons Attribution License (http://creativecommons.org/licenses/by/3.0), which permits unrestricted use, distribution, and reproduction in any medium, provided the original work is properly cited.

References

[1] Adler Y, Charron P, Imazio M, Badano L, Barón-Esquivias G, Bogaert J, et al. 2015 ESC guidelines for the diagnosis and management of pericardial diseases: The TaskForce for the Diagnosis and Management of Pericardial Diseases of the European Society of Cardiology (ESC) endorsed by: The European Association for Cardio-Thoracic Surgery (EACTS). European Heart Journal. 2015;**36**(42):2921-2964. DOI: 10.1093/eurheartj/ehv318

[2] Imazio M. Contemporary management of pericardial diseases. Current Opinion in Cardiology. 2012;**27**(3):308-317. DOI: 10.1097/HCO.0b013e3283524fbe

[3] Klein AL, Abbara S, Agler DA, Appleton CP, Asher CR, Hoit B, et al. American society of echocardiography clinical recommendations for multimodality cardiovascular imaging of patients with pericardial disease: Endorsed by the society for cardiovascular magnetic resonance and society of cardiovascular computed tomography. Journal of the American Society of Echocardiography. 2013;**26**(9):965-1012. DOI: 10.1016/j.echo.2013.06.023

[4] Maisch B, Ristić AD, Pankuweit S. Intrapericardial treatment of autoreactive pericardial effusion with triamcinolone: The way to avoid side effects of systemic corticosteroid therapy. European Heart Journal. 2002;**23**(19):1503-1508

[5] Frasiolas JA, Cahoon WD. Intrapericardial triamcinolone administration for autoreactive pericarditis. The Annals of Pharmacotherapy. 2010;**44**(10):1641-1646. DOI: 10.1345/aph.1P294

[6] Murashita T, Schaff HV, Daly RC, Oh JK, Dearani JA, Stulak JM, et al. Experience with pericardiectomy for constrictive pericarditis over eight decades. The Annals of Thoracic Surgery. 2017;**104**(3):742-750. DOI: 10.1016/j.athoracsur.2017.05.063

Chapter 2

Pericardial Diseases in Elderly Patients

Ammar Athar, Kartik Dhaduk and Wilbert S. Aronow

Abstract

The pericardium is a double-walled, fibrous sac typically containing 20–50 mL of fluid surrounding the heart and great vessels. In addition to its known anatomical and physiological functions, the pericardium also serves an active immunological role that is the focus of interest pertaining to inflammatory cardiac conditions such as pericarditis and myocarditis. In the geriatric population, the pericardium also undergoes age-related changes similar to other anatomical structures; however, in contrast to common cardiac diseases such as coronary artery disease, heart failure, valvular disease, etc., data from randomized trials regarding the management of pericardial diseases are limited, especially in the elderly population. In this chapter, we will discuss age-related pericardial anatomical changes, various pericardial diseases (acute, recurrent and constrictive pericarditis, pericardial effusion, cardiac tamponade, etc.) along with their clinical impact, and evidence-based management.

Keywords: pericardial disease, elderly, acute pericarditis, constrictive pericarditis, recurrent pericarditis, cardiac tamponade, pericardium, myocarditis

1. Age-related pericardial anatomical changes

The pericardium is subject to age-related changes just like any other organ in the human body although available literature regarding pericardial anatomy and pericardial disease etiology related to aging is very limited. One study examining bovine pericardium for age-dependent differences in collagen alignment showed higher elasticity, higher tensile strength, and thin pericardium in neonatal compared to adult bovine pericardium [1]. Despite such noted anatomical changes in the pericardial structure with age, the spectrum of pericardial disease remains similar among younger and older populations. Although most guidelines have not discussed specific age-related pericardial disease management, diagnostic evaluation and treatment of pericarditis in the geriatric population should take comorbidities into consideration for optimal management [2].

2. Pericardial effusion

The pericardial space contains 20–50 mL of fluid in the pericardial sac which works as a lubricant between two layers of pericardium. Pericardial effusion is defined by an excess fluid collection over the normal physiological amount within this space. Pericardial fluid accumulation can be secondary to increased fluid production (i.e., any inflammatory condition) or from reduced fluid reabsorption (i.e., heart failure, pulmonary hypertension, and pericardial lymphatic obstruction). The fluid starts accumulating according to gravitational forces, initially in the posterior-inferior site then circumferentially resulting in moderate to large effusion.

Pericardial effusion can be classified based on various characteristics such as size (mild, moderate, and large), onset (acute, subacute, and chronic), distribution (localized or circumferential), composition (transudate, exudate, blood, or rarely gas from bacterial infections), and hemodynamic effects (without tamponade, with tamponade, effusive-constrictive) [2, 3]. (**Table 1**).

The normal pericardium is made up of a high content of collagen fibers, which creates a relatively inelastic sac that contains the heart. The pressure-volume curve of the normal pericardium is a J-shaped curve, which allows a limited stretch of the pericardium in response to physiological events such as posture or volume status without significant change in the intrapericardial pressure; however, after reaching a certain intrapericardial volume, the intrapericardial pressure rises suddenly and can cause sudden systemic hemodynamic derangements. The rapid rate of the fluid collection also plays a role in the pressure-volume curve; a sudden rise in intrapericardial volume (such as with aortic dissection or trauma with hemopericardium) of 100–200 mL significantly raises the intrapericardial pressure, whereas the slow collection of fluid may allow the development of a large pericardial effusion (1–2 L) without signs of cardiac tamponade [3, 4].

2.1 Etiology

Among the elderly, the spectrum of etiologies for pericardial effusion does not differ significantly from the rest of the population. The underlying cause of effusion can usually be inferred from the clinical picture. One study in 322 patients

Size of fluid collection in TTE*	Less than 10 mm—mild
	10–20 mm—moderate
	More than 20 mm—large
Onset of fluid collection	<1 week—acute
	>1 week to <3 months—subacute
	>3 months—chronic
Fluid distribution	Localized
	Circumferential
Fluid composition	Infectious—exudative Non-infectious—transudate
	Hemopericardium—blood
	Pneumopericardium—air
	Chylopericardium—chylous
Hemodynamic effects	No tamponade effect
	Tamponade effect
	effusive-constrictive

**TTE, transthoracic echocardiography.*

Table 1.
Classification of pericardial effusion.

has reported around 60% of cases had a known cause of pericardial effusion [5]. A varying amount of effusion can be seen in other conditions such as malignancy (with or without direct pericardial involvement), renal failure, pregnancy, aortic or cardiac wall rupture, trauma, heart failure, cirrhosis of the liver, nephrotic syndrome, autoimmune diseases, radiation, etc. One study incorporated demographics in their review of pericarditis etiology by comparing a younger patient population (age 15–65, n = 221) to a geriatric population (age 66–88, n = 101) and found no statistically significant differences in the incidence of idiopathic (33 vs. 38%) versus neoplastic (14.4 vs. 10.8%) pericarditis or the incidence of tamponade (36 vs. 38.6%) [6]. The cause of effusion may also vary by geographical area and clinical setting. For example, effusions related to viral pericarditis or idiopathic pericarditis are more common in outpatient populations of the western world, whereas bacterial and tuberculous inflammation and effusion are more common in sub-Saharan Africa and the developing world. Effusions associated with uremic pericarditis or malignancies are frequently found in hospital settings [3, 7].

According to one study with a mean participant age of 56, when determining the cause of moderate to severe pleural effusions, it is important to consider three major factors: (1) size of effusion; (2) presence of tamponade; and (3) inflammatory signs (defined as two or more from: fever >37°C, pericardial friction rub, characteristic chest pain, and diffuse ST-segment elevation). The presence of inflammatory signs was associated with acute idiopathic pericarditis (likelihood ratio = 5.4, $P < 0.001$), a large effusion without any inflammatory signs or tamponade was found to be associated with chronic idiopathic pericardial effusion (likelihood ratio = 20, $P < 0.001$), and the features of tamponade without inflammatory signs were associated with malignant effusions (likelihood ratio = 2.9, $P < 0.01$) [5].

2.2 Clinical presentation

The presentation of pericardial effusion varies according to the speed of accumulation, size of effusion, and etiology. The rate of fluid collection plays a critical role in clinical presentation as rapidly accumulating pericardial effusion causes a quick rise in intrapericardial pressure, which results in cardiac tamponade, while slowly accumulating fluid accommodates comparatively larger volume before signs of tamponade [2, 3]. The cases of isolated pericardial effusion can be asymptomatic or can have symptoms related to the underlying etiology or to the effusion itself. The classically reported symptom is dyspnea on exertion; however, the wide spectrum of symptoms related to compressive effect includes cough, weakness, fatigue, palpitations (from compressive effect of the pericardial fluid or reduced blood pressure), nausea (diaphragm), dysphagia (esophagus), hoarseness of voice (recurrent laryngeal nerve), etc. Patients may present with fever from underlying disease (infectious or systemic inflammatory disease), pleural effusion, ascites, or hepatic dysfunction from long standing pericardial constriction [2, 8].

Physical examination may remain normal without any significant findings in patients with no hemodynamic compromise. Pulsus paradoxus is an inspiratory drop in systolic BP >10 mmHg due to the augmentation of right ventricular preload causing impaired left ventricular filling resulting in abnormal decrease in stroke volume [9] and is a phenomenon commonly seen with large pericardial effusion or cardiac tamponade. Pericardial friction rub is rarely heard but is a usual finding of pericarditis.

2.3 Diagnostics

Upon clinical suspicion of pericardial effusion, the diagnostic approach should consider three major steps: (1) confirm the presence of effusion; (2)

assess the hemodynamic impact; and (3) effort to identify the underlying etiology. Transthoracic echocardiography (TTE) is recommended in all patients with suspected effusion as a class I, level C recommendation. Further imaging modalities such as computed tomography (CT) scan, cardiac magnetic resonance imaging (CMRI), pericardial fluid analysis, or biopsy can be considered in cases where loculated effusion, masses, or thickening of the pericardium are suspected. Basic diagnostic work up, including blood counts, chemistry, thyroid function tests, cardiac biomarkers, inflammatory markers such as C-reactive protein (CRP) and sedimentation rate (ESR), electrocardiogram (ECG), and chest X-ray, should be done [2, 10]. ECG findings in pericardial effusion include low QRS voltage and electrical alternans, a finding of large pericardial effusion or tamponade that is usually associated with sinus tachycardia.

TTE is recommended as the first modality to determine the hemodynamic significance of pericardial effusion and is highly sensitive and specific. The pericardial fluid appears as echo-lucent space between the pericardium and epicardium on TTE. The semi-quantitative assessment for largest echo-free space in echocardiographic views provides an assessment of severity. Mild pericardial effusion is considered <10 mm, moderate between 10 and 20 mm, and large effusion is any collection >20 mm. The collection of effusion follows gravity initially in the inferolateral position close to right atrium in the apical four chamber view with the patient in a supine-left lateral position. The pattern of collection changes to circumferential in the pericardium with increasing amount of fluid (**Figure 1**). After the development of a large amount of effusion, the heart can be seen swinging in the pericardial cavity, a finding that correlates with electrical alternans on ECG [2, 3, 11].

Cardiac CT and CMRI are useful imaging modalities for the evaluation of pericardial effusion and tamponade especially for more detailed assessment and the localization of the effusion and associated abnormalities in the mediastinum, lungs,

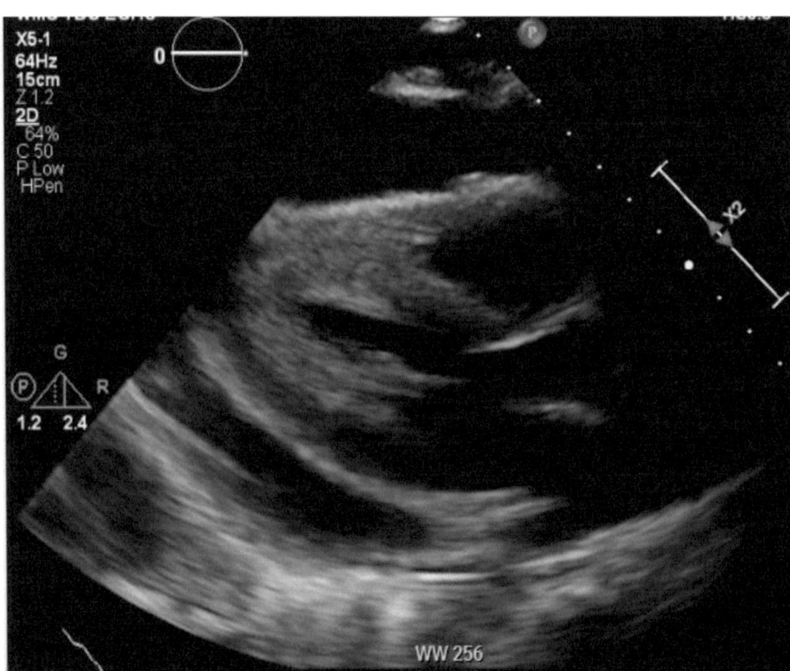

Figure 1.
Large circumferential pericardial effusion.

and adjacent structures. They are useful for the guidance of pericardiocentesis since loculated effusions or calcified pericardium can be identified. CMRI is superior to CT in differentiating fluids especially highly exudative fluid from thickened pericardium. CT detects a minimum amount of pericardial calcium and is relatively quick [2, 11].

Pericardial fluid analysis is often performed when the patient requires pericardiocentesis. Routine fluid studies include measuring fluid protein level, protein fluid/serum ratio, lactate dehydrogenase (LDH), LDH fluid/serum ratio, glucose, cell counts, and specific gravity. Fluid cytology and tumor markers (carcinoembryonic antigen, cancer antigen 19-9, adenosine deaminase, and interferon gamma) are useful measures in malignancy. Polymerase chain reaction and fluid cultures help in infectious etiologies.

2.4 Treatment

For small-to-medium sized, asymptomatic pericardial effusion without signs of hemodynamic instability, regular outpatient follow-up with clinical examination and/or echocardiography should be preferred. Management of pericardial effusion with signs of inflammation (pericarditis) should follow the standard or treatment for pericarditis; however, in the absence of any inflammation, anti-inflammatory drugs, such as nonsteroidal anti-inflammatory drugs (NSAIDs), colchicine, and corticosteroids, are generally not effective. Such cases as well as cases with large effusion that failed empiric anti-inflammatory therapy would require pericardiocentesis. Recurrence of effusion is fairly common and further management options include pericardial window formation or pericardiectomy. A study comparing patients age 15–65 to a group of patients age 66–88 years showed elderly people had more persistence of effusion (6.3 vs. 14%; $P < 0.05$) but no statistically significant difference in mortality (24 vs. 30%) or evolution of cardiac constriction (4 vs. 2%) during median follow up time of 11 months [6]. There is no standard guideline available for elderly patients regarding pleural effusions; however, the expert consensus suggests adjusting the type and dosages of medications with special attention to drug interactions and renal function given the prevalence of polypharmacy and renal dysfunction in the geriatric population [2]. A proposed management algorithm for pericardial effusion of unknown origin is depicted in **Figure 2** [2, 3].

2.5 Prognosis

The prognosis of pericardial effusion is related to its etiology and size. Moderate-to-large size effusions are more commonly associated with bacterial infection, systemic inflammatory disease, or malignancy. Idiopathic pericardial effusion has a good prognosis, but effusion related to bacteria, post-radiation, or pericardial injury has a higher rate of developing either early (cardiac tamponade) or late complications (constrictive pericarditis). Large effusion (>3 months) carries a 30–35% risk of progression to cardiac tamponade. The follow-up of pericardial effusion is mainly based on symptomatic evaluation with the follow-up of inflammatory biomarkers and echocardiography [3]. A recent meta-analysis regarding prognosis of pericardial effusion in an elderly population with mean age > 60 reported that pericardial effusion can be considered as a marker of severity of the underlying disease as evidenced by a higher hazard ratio (HR) in patients with pericardial effusion with myocardial infarction (HR 2.65, 95% CI: 1.4–4.99; $P = 0.003$, 15 months follow-up) versus those with chronic heart failure (HR 1.53, 95% CI: 1.22–1.92; $P < 0.0001$, 31 months follow-up) [12].

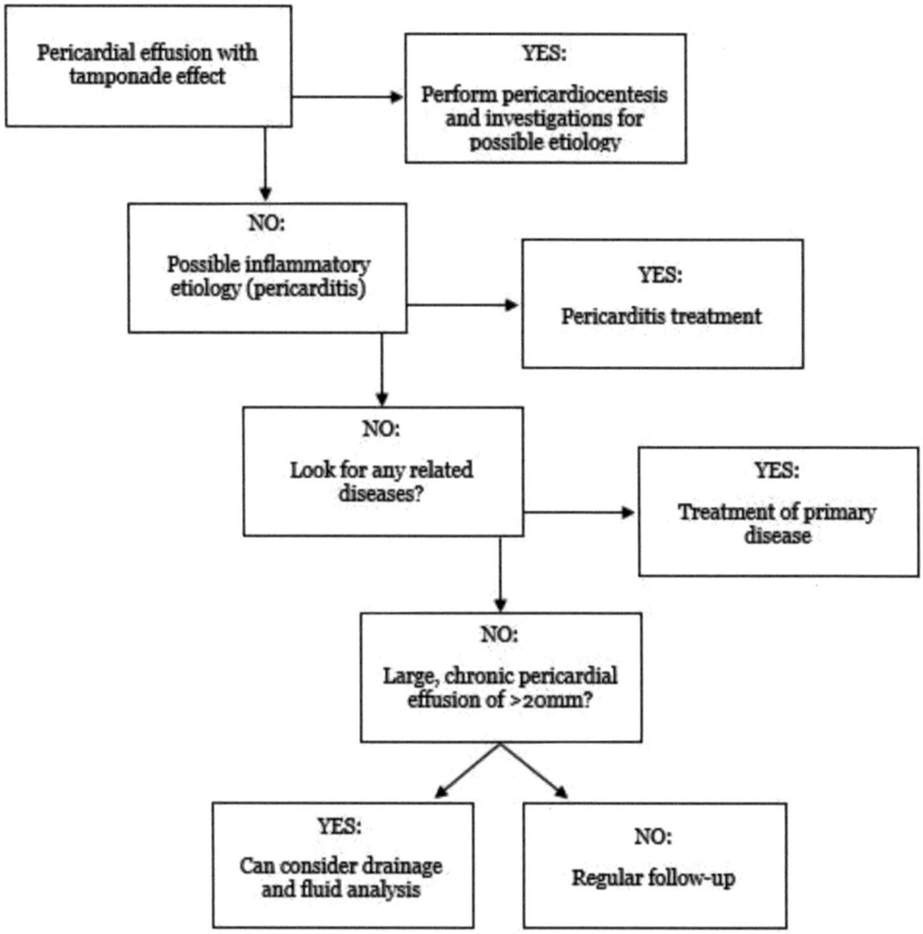

Figure 2.
Management algorithm for pericardial effusion with unknown origin.

3. Acute pericarditis

Acute pericarditis is a condition defined by the inflammation of the pericardial sac that can take place in the setting of a systemic disease (infectious, malignant, inflammatory, etc.) or independently of any other condition [2, 5, 13–15]. Among the elderly, it is important to consider malignancy in the evaluation of etiology as it is more common in this population and may prompt appropriate testing leading to a faster diagnosis and potential earlier intervention.

3.1 Etiology

Various infections (viral, bacterial, fungal, and tick-borne) have been known to cause the inflammation of the pericardium. In fact, prior to the widespread distribution of anti-retroviral medications, pericarditis was found to be the most common cardiovascular manifestation of human immunodeficiency virus/acquired immunodeficiency syndrome [16, 17] and, in conjunction with tuberculosis, remains the most common cause of pericardial inflammation in the developing world [18], whereas coxsackievirus maintains its status as the most common viral etiology of pericarditis overall. Malignancy, independent of other systemic diseases, has also been associated with acute pericardial disease and accounts for about 6% of cases without another explanation [19, 20]. Systemic diseases, such as systemic lupus erythematosus (SLE) and rheumatoid arthritis (RA), have been found to cause pericardial inflammation with approximately 50% of patients with SLE experiencing pericarditis. Other established etiologies of acute pericardial disease include post-myocardial infarction pericardial inflammation and/or effusion [21–24], post-radiation pericarditis with or without pericardial effusion [25], and uremic pericarditis usually in the setting of advanced renal failure and inadequate dialysis [26, 27]. Hypothyroidism severe enough to result in myxedema can result in a large, slowly accumulating pericardial effusion but rarely causes acute pericarditis [28].

3.2 Clinical presentation

There are four major distinctive features of acute pericarditis (at least two of which are required to make a clinical diagnosis): chest pain, pericardial friction rub, characteristic ECG changes, and pericardial effusion. The predominant presenting symptom is chest pain that is usually pleuritic in nature, sharp and alleviated by sitting up and leaning forward due to the positional shift of the pericardium, a feature which distinguishes it from the typical chest pain caused by myocardial ischemia [29, 30]. Pericardial chest pain is also often associated with nonproductive cough and dyspnea [29]. A scratchy, squeaking sound heard over the left sternal border upon auscultation known as a pericardial friction rub is the second of four major clinical features of pericarditis and is reported to be found in approximately 85% of patients with acute pericarditis in the absence of a pericardial effusion [20]. It is an extra heart sound resulting from the friction between the parietal and visceral pericardium coming into contact in the presence of inflammation. The presence of a pericardial effusion is the third of the four major signs of acute pericarditis and can best be appreciated on an echocardiogram. The last of the four major signs of pericarditis is new, diffuse ST-elevation, PR segment depressions, and PR segment elevation in lead aVR found on ECG (discussed further under *Diagnostics*) [15, 29, 31]. Other secondary features of pericarditis that may or may not be present are fever, subacute course of chest pain, elevated troponin (suggestive of myocardial involvement), and hemodynamic instability (suggestive of cardiac tamponade) [32, 33].

3.3 Diagnostics

Various laboratory tests and imaging modalities play role in establishing the diagnosis of acute pericarditis. Inflammatory markers, such as white blood cell count (WBC), erythrocyte sedimentation rate (ESR), and C-reactive protein (CRP) levels although nonspecific, may help distinguish pericarditis from a condition with overlapping features given appropriate clinical criteria. Troponin levels, usually elevated in acute coronary syndrome, may also be elevated in pericarditis indicating myocardial involvement [34].

The chest X-ray may show cardiomegaly in the presence of a significant pericardial effusion but otherwise has limited utility in the diagnosis of pericardial disease. An echocardiogram can be similarly useful although the absence of pericardial effusion would not necessarily exclude the diagnosis of acute pericarditis. Cardiac CT imaging can serve a dual purpose in the diagnosis of acute pericarditis in that it may also help elucidate the underlying pathology responsible for the inflammatory changes. Pericardial thickening and effusion in the absence of calcification along with the enhancement of the visceral and parietal pericardium with intravenous contrast are indicative of active inflammation consistent with pericarditis [35]. CMRI can confirm inflammation but is likely not necessary in the diagnostic workup of acute pericarditis unless the presumed etiology is a systemic inflammatory or autoimmune disease with characteristic cardiac findings.

The ECG may be perhaps the most useful diagnostic modality when considering acute pericarditis. The ECG progresses through a distinctive, four stage pattern although the evolution can be variable with up to 40% of patients showing atypical changes [30–32]. Stage 1 is characterized by widespread ST elevation with reciprocal ST depression in leads aVR and V1 as well as PR segment elevation in lead aVR accompanied by PR segment depression in the remaining limb leads and V5–6. Within 1 week of onset, normalization of ST and PR segments on the ECG comprises Stage 2. Stage 3 of the ECG is marked by diffuse T-wave inversions, while Stage 4 consists of normalization of the ECG. However, not all forms of pericarditis result in the characteristic ECG pattern as the pericardium itself is an inert tissue and only inflammatory changes involving the epicardium or myocardium would be reflected in acute pericarditis [36]. In fact, one review found that of 100 patients studied, only seven arrhythmias were identified all resulting from underlying heart disease [37], while a separate study comparing acute pericarditis to myopericarditis found arrhythmias more frequently associated with myopericarditis [38].

3.4 Treatment

Medical treatment of acute pericarditis utilizes one or a combination of two out of three different medications: NSAIDs, colchicine, and glucocorticoids. Treatment duration is usually guided by the resolution of symptoms and etiology of disease in the absence of confounding factors such as acute kidney or liver injury.

A combination of NSAIDs and colchicine is the mainstay of therapy for acute viral or idiopathic pericarditis. NSAIDs alone have been shown through multiple studies to effectively treat up to 80% of pericarditis cases [20, 32, 39]. No one particular NSAIDs has been shown to be more effective than another except in the case of post-myocardial infarction pericarditis for which aspirin is recommended and other NSAIDs should be avoided in order to prevent the disruption of myocardial scar formation [40]. Patients taking NSAIDs for pericarditis should concurrently take a proton-pump inhibitor for ulcer prophylaxis in the absence of any direct contraindication to do so. Treatment can be tapered once the patient is symptom-free for at least 24 hours (typically 1–2 weeks). Alternatively, one study recommends following weekly CRP levels along with symptom resolution and beginning tapering, once the patient is symptom-free for 24 hours and CRP levels have returned to normal [41].

In 2005, the Colchicine for Acute Pericarditis (COPE) trial suggested colchicine as an effective adjunct for treating acute pericarditis when combined with NSAIDs therapy for patients with non-bacterial, non-malignancy-related pericardial disease [39]. The addition of colchicine was further shown to reduce symptom burden and decrease the rate of recurrent pericarditis by a subsequent, randomized-control trial (RCT) [42], a finding, which was later supported by a meta-analysis in 2014, that demonstrated a reduced risk of recurrence at 18 months in patients undergoing treatment for acute pericarditis [43]. The management of acute pericarditis with a combination of NSAIDs and colchicine is also currently supported by the 2015 European Society of Cardiology (ESC) guidelines [2].

For patients with contraindications to NSAIDs therapy (kidney failure, GI bleeding, pregnancy, etc.), glucocorticoids may be used in combination with colchicine for the initial treatment of acute pericarditis. Treatment duration is then guided by symptom resolution and the normalization of CRP levels with tapering usually started 2–4 weeks thereafter. Glucocorticoids have also been utilized in patients with pericarditis refractory to NSAIDs and colchicine though one study shows a trend toward higher rate of recurrent pericarditis with steroid use [44].

Geriatric patients appear to have a higher risk of mortality when admitted and treated for pericarditis in the hospital. Although data regarding treatment of specifically elderly patients are sparse, one study examined the relationship between pericarditis, age, hospital admission, and mortality. They analyzed 45,504 patients above the age of 65 from 1999 to 2012 and found that hospitalization for the treatment of pericarditis is associated with increased risk of 1-year all-cause mortality despite a decrease in 1-year mortality rate from 19.7% (95% confidence interval (CI) 18.8–20.8) in 1999 to 17.3% (95% CI 15.3–20) in 2012 [45]. While it is possible that this association is in part due to a higher prevalence of significant comorbidities and compromised immune systems among the elderly, it nevertheless remains an aspect of pericardial disease that warrants further investigation as advanced therapies and support devices continue to enable longer lifespans with time.

4. Recurrent pericarditis

Recurrent pericarditis is a syndrome defined by the reemergence of pericarditis after the treatment of the initial inflammatory event [31, 46–48]. A minimum 4–6 week symptom-free interval post anti-inflammatory treatment is required to differentiate recurrent pericarditis from incessant pericarditis.

4.1 Etiology

Acute pericarditis has been found to have recurrence rates as high as 30% in patients treated without colchicine [32, 39, 47, 49]. Some cases of recurrent pericarditis appear to reflect localized inflammation given the detection of certain cytokines (interleukin (IL)-6, IL-8, and interferon gamma) in the pericardial fluid and their absence in the serum [50]; however, most cases are considered to be of autoimmune etiology [2, 51].

4.2 Clinical presentation

Chest pain appears to be the most common recurring symptom; however, the clinical diagnosis of recurrent pericarditis requires the presence of at least one of the following in addition to pleuritic chest pain: fever, pericardial rub, ECG changes, pericardial effusion, elevated WBC, ESR, CRP, or evidence of active pericardial inflammation on imaging [15]. Patients with previously treated pericarditis may experience multiple recurrences over the course of months to years following the initial event [52–54].

4.3 Diagnostics

The selection of the initial treatment regimen can directly impact the potential for the recurrence of acute pericarditis and may serve as an independent predictor of risk. For instance, a prior response to NSAIDs therapy is associated with the reduced risk of recurrence [32], whereas treatment with glucocorticoids is associated with increased recurrence [55]. It is difficult to rely upon ECG changes for the diagnosis for recurrent pericarditis as they are non-specific in the majority of cases. Chest X-ray and TTE also have limited utility as both will appear to be normal without a significant pericardial effusion. CT and CMRI imaging have proven to be of benefit in elucidating the diagnosis of recurrent pericarditis as contrast-enhanced CT can detect active pericardial inflammation while CMRI may reveal the evidence of edema via pericardial gadolinium enhancement [2, 35].

4.4 Treatment

Recurrent viral or idiopathic pericarditis is typically managed with an outpatient medical regimen [2, 52, 54] initially consisting of an NSAIDs and colchicine [15] as glucocorticoids are known to increase the risk of recurrence despite multiple recurrences of pericarditis [56]. Glucocorticoid therapy is, therefore, reserved for patients who are either unable to tolerate NSAIDs or have failed NSAIDs therapy in the past [2].

It is important to ensure an adequate trial of NSAIDs was given prior to labeling a patient as refractory. Common agents such as Aspirin and Ibuprofen should be attempted first followed by Indomethacin for treatment resistant cases. Medication should be administered in three doses over 24 hours to ensure consistent therapeutic levels, and dosage should be titrated up as needed to achieve symptom control until the daily maximum is reached or symptoms have subsided [10, 32, 39, 52, 54, 57].

Patients with recurrent pericarditis are often times designated as refractory to colchicine therapy after having received inappropriate dosing or rapid tapers [43]. In addition, colchicine should be given twice a day in order to reduce the risk of poor compliance due to gastrointestinal discomfort [10, 57, 58].

In cases of recurrent pericarditis refractory to treatment with NSAIDs, colchicine, and glucocorticoids, patients found to have the evidence of systemic inflammation may benefit from anti-interleukin-1 therapy. A recent trial in 2016 demonstrated a significant reduction of recurrence (90–18%) in patients with pericarditis resistant to colchicine and dependent on corticosteroids with the addition of anakinra, an IL-1B antagonist [59]. Although promising, this study's results were limited by a small sample size and inconsistent colchicine dosing across trial participants warranting further investigation.

5. Constrictive pericarditis

Constrictive pericarditis is a condition that occurs when a thickened or calcified pericardium loses elasticity resulting in the reduction of diastolic filling. It is a syndrome that is the end result of chronic pericarditis and pericardial effusion gradually progressing to fibrosis [2, 15, 29, 60]. Such impairment overtime causes the reduction of pericardial space, which in turn uncouples intrathoracic and intracardiac pressures generating increased interventricular interdependence visible on echocardiogram [2, 35, 61, 62].

5.1 Etiology

Constrictive pericarditis can occur as a result of inflammation and effusion from any pericardial disease [2, 31, 63]. A combination of studies has found that 42 to 61% of cases were idiopathic or viral, 11 to 37% postcardiac surgery, 2 to 31% postradiation, 3 to 7% due to connective tissue disorders, 3 to 15% bacterial or tuberculous, and 1 to 10% related to malignancy, trauma, drug toxicity, sarcoidosis, or uremic pericarditis [64–69]. Tuberculosis remains a major global cause of constrictive pericarditis especially in endemic nations [2, 70].

5.2 Clinical presentation

Patients with constrictive pericarditis usually present with symptoms of right heart failure in the absence of ventricular function impairment. Symptoms are consistent with volume overload, such as edema, pleural effusion, dyspnea, ascites, or low output states such as exertional dyspnea and fatigue [2]. As high as 93% of patients present with elevated jugular venous pressure (JVP) [65], while only approximately 20% of patients present with pulsus paradoxus or Kussmaul's sign [64, 65, 71]. A pericardial knock has been noted in 47% of patients with constrictive pericarditis [65].

5.3 Diagnostics

Although the diagnosis of constrictive pericarditis can be made by echocardiography [72], an ECG and chest X-ray should also be obtained as part of the initial evaluation. There are no specific ECG changes consistently indicative of constrictive pericarditis; however, an ECG may be helpful in ruling out other cardiac pathology. The chest X-ray may show the evidence of pericardial calcification in which the presence of right heart failure would be strongly suggestive of constrictive pericarditis; however, the absence of such a finding would not rule out the disease [2].

All patients with suspected pericardial disease should be evaluated with echocardiography [2, 73]. Septal bounce and pericardial thickening on M-mode and 2-dimensional echocardiography would be suggestive of a constrictive pattern. On Doppler echocardiography, increased interventricular interdependence is associated with pericardial fibrosis, and the ratio of the right ventricular (RV) area to the left ventricular (LV) area, known as systolic area index (SAI), is virtually diagnostic of constrictive pericarditis when the SAI is >1.1 [74].

CT imaging can show pericardial thickening and calcification but is not necessary to diagnose constrictive pericarditis. However, the identification of important vascular structures on CT can prove useful if planning for pericardiectomy [75]. Positron emission tomography (PET)/CT can also be helpful in predicting response to corticosteroid therapy [76]. CMRI may show characteristic changes of constrictive pericarditis, such as pericardial thickening, dilation of the inferior vena cava, or ventricular interdependence, but is usually necessary unless investigating other related cardiac pathology.

5.4 Treatment

Treatment of constrictive pericarditis is dependent on the course of the disease at the time of evaluation. For early subacute disease in patients who are hemodynamically stable, medical therapy similar to that used for acute pericarditis is recommended. Patients who present with the evidence of late chronic disease (cachexia, pericardial calcifications, and hepatic dysfunction) or those who have failed conservative management with anti-inflammatory therapy can be treated with pericardiectomy [63]. The majority of patients achieve symptomatic relief with early surgical removal of the inflamed pericardium [69] with one study reporting up to 69% of patients being symptom-free at 4 year follow-up [65].

6. Cardiac tamponade

Cardiac tamponade is characterized by the accumulation of pericardial fluid causing significant impairment in cardiac function due to the pressure effect of external pericardial content causing compression of all cardiac chambers. Increase in intrapericardial pressure reduces the myocardial transmural pressure with a reduced ventricular wall diastolic compliance and a decrease in cardiac output and blood pressure. In cardiac tamponade, unlike constrictive pericarditis, most of the inspiratory decline in the intrathoracic pressure is transmitted through the pericardium to the right ventricle and results in increased venous return and right ventricular distention. The higher intrapericardial pressure limits the right ventricular free wall expansion, resulting in bulging of the right ventricular septum to the left ventricle. This bulge diminishes the compliance of the left ventricle, which results in decreased filling and cardiac output [4, 77]. A similar mechanism contributes to pulsus paradoxus, an abnormal decline in systolic blood pressure (>10 mmHg) with inspiration. Cardiac tamponade is a treatable cause of cardiogenic shock that can be rapidly fatal.

Usually, cardiac tamponade is seen after pericarditis, tuberculosis, iatrogenic (secondary to cardiac interventions), trauma, neoplasm, with other uncommon causes including, collagen vascular disorder, radiation therapy, post-myocardial infarction, uremia, aortic dissection, and a bacterial infection.

6.1 Etiology

Cardiac tamponade could be acute, subacute, low-pressure type, or regional. Acute cardiac tamponade is sudden in onset and acutely life-threatening if not treated. Subacute cardiac tamponade is less dramatic compared to acute, but once the intrapericardial pressure reaches the threshold, patients experience classical tamponade symptoms related to decreased cardiac function. Low-pressure tamponade is a condition that appears in hypovolemic patients (such as traumatic hemorrhage, over diuresis, etc.). Correction of volume status reveals a typical tamponade pattern. Regional tamponade occurs from loculated effusion or a localized hematoma causing compression of only selected chambers. It is usually seen after myocardial infarction or pericardiotomy [77].

6.2 Clinical presentation

Depending on the severity of the tamponade, a variety of clinical findings are seen. Sinus tachycardia as a physiologic response to maintain the cardiac output is common. Elevated jugular venous pressure, muffled heart sounds, and systemic hypotension together referred to as Beck's triad is a pathognomonic sign for tamponade.

6.3 Diagnosis

The diagnostic approach and the evaluation of cardiac tamponade are similar to that for patients with suspected pericardial effusion. The ECG findings include sinus tachycardia, low voltage of QRS complex, and frequently electrical alternans, which is beat-to-beat changes in the position of the heart with relation to cardiac tamponade. The presence of total electrical alternans, including P wave, QRS complex, and ST segment alternans, is highly specific for cardiac tamponade, but sensitivity is very low with findings present in only 5–10% of cases. The presence of lone QRS alternans is more common but is not very specific for tamponade. The presence of QRS vector alternans (axis shift) is more specific than QRS amplitude alternans for the cardiac tamponade [77, 78].

TTE is the standard first-line imaging technique recommended for the evaluation of cardiac tamponade with excellent safety and efficacy. The size of the pericardial effusion does not indicate significance. Since respiration has an impact on intracardiac pressures, mainly on the right side of the heart, this respirophasic flow pattern becomes more evident in tamponade, which can be measured by Doppler echocardiographic variations in blood flow across the mitral (>25% variation) (**Figure 3**) and tricuspid valves (>40% variation) as well as pulmonary and systemic outflow. Right atrial collapse and RV collapse on diastole (**Figure 4**) are usual signs of cardiac tamponade, but in the setting of severe pulmonary hypertension, right-sided chamber collapse may be delayed and preceded by left atrial collapse. In most cases, the thickness of the left ventricular wall and lower compliance prevents LV collapse. As the tamponade worsens, there are progressive impairments in hemodynamics and intracardiac flows. Elevated pressures in the right atrium can

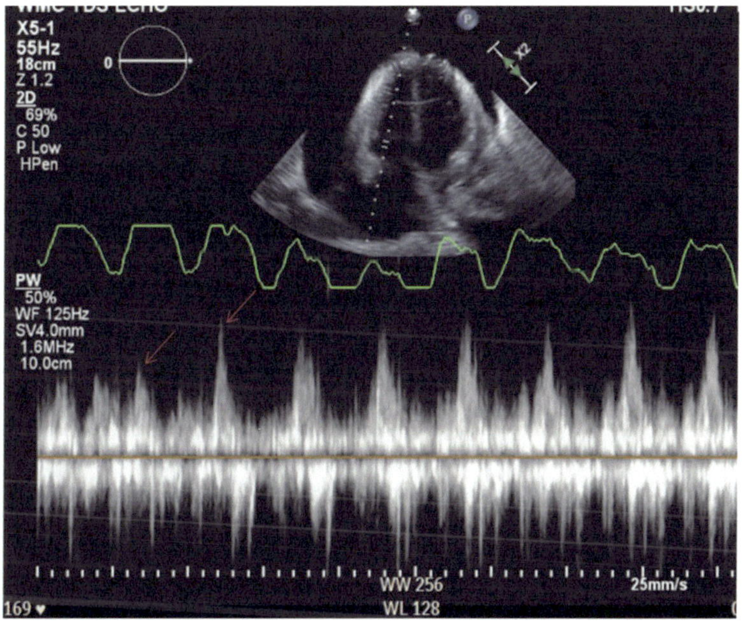

Figure 3.
Doppler echocardiographic variations in blood flow across the mitral valve.

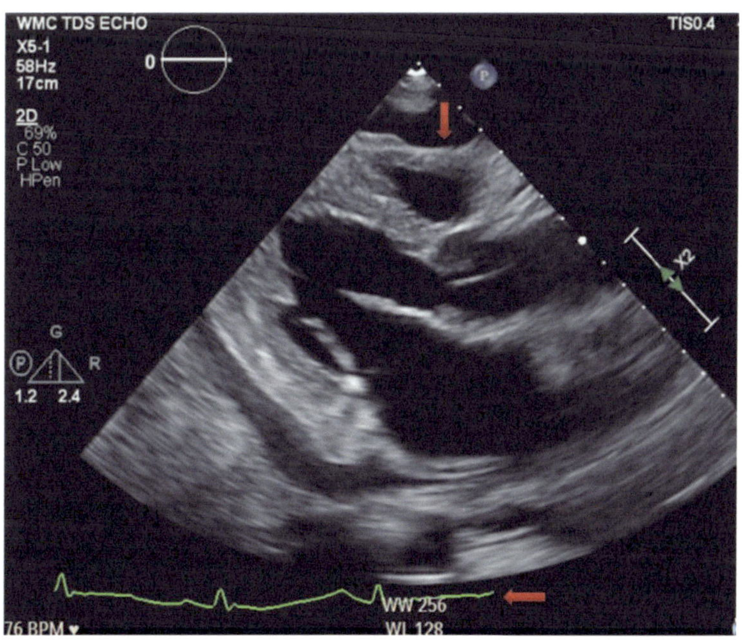

Figure 4.
Diastolic collapse of the right ventricular wall (top arrow) and diastolic period of cardiac cycle (bottom arrow).

be assessed from a plethora of the inferior vena cava (IVC) which is a lack of change in IVC caliber in response to respiratory flow pattern (<50% reduction in IVC diameter during inspiration). The swinging movement of the heart within the pericardial sac is another echocardiographic sign. These TTE findings in cardiac structural and functional change with a decline in cardiac function often occur well before the onset of pulsus paradoxus and significant clinical deterioration, and thus, they are an important indicator in cardiac tamponade [11, 79]. Cardiac CT and CMRI may provide valuable information about the functional and structural change of the heart and pericardium, but they are only required in special conditions such as localized tamponade, loculated pericardial effusion, or hematoma [61, 79].

6.4 Treatment

The treatment of cardiac tamponade is decompression with pericardiocentesis which can be done by percutaneous catheter pericardiocentesis or open surgical drainage with or without a pericardial window or video-assisted thoracoscopic pericardiectomy. Catheter pericardiocentesis under echocardiographic or fluoroscopic guidance is a more rapid and less invasive technique. Surgical pericardiocentesis is usually performed in purulent pericarditis bleeding into the pericardium or when pericardial biopsies and pericardiectomy are needed [2, 77]. A triage system proposed by the ESC Working Group on Myocardial and Pericardial Diseases can be used to guide the timing of the pericardiocentesis in non-emergent cases [80]. Fluid removal and decompression of the pericardial cavity rapidly improve the clinical hemodynamic status. Positive pressure mechanical ventilation should be avoided as it increases the intrathoracic pressure that deteriorates cardiac filling. The use of vasodilators and diuretics that reduce the preload is not recommended in the presence of cardiac tamponade [2].

Disclosure

None of the authors have any conflicts of interest to disclose.

Author details

Ammar Athar†, Kartik Dhaduk† and Wilbert S. Aronow*
Cardiology Division, Department of Medicine, Westchester Medical Center and New York Medical College, NY, USA

*Address all correspondence to: wsaronow@aol.com

† These authors are contributed equally.

IntechOpen

© 2019 The Author(s). Licensee IntechOpen. This chapter is distributed under the terms of the Creative Commons Attribution License (http://creativecommons.org/licenses/by/3.0), which permits unrestricted use, distribution, and reproduction in any medium, provided the original work is properly cited.

References

[1] Sizeland KH, Wells HC, Higgins J, Cunanan CM, Kirby N, Hawley A, et al. Age dependent differences in collagen alignment of glutaraldehyde fixed bovine pericardium. BioMed Research International. 2014;**2014**:189197

[2] Adler Y, Charron P, Imazio M, Badano L, Baron-Esquivias G, Bogaert J, et al. 2015 ESC guidelines for the diagnosis and management of pericardial diseases: The task force for the diagnosis and Management of Pericardial Diseases of the European Society of Cardiology (ESC) endorsed by: The European Association for Cardio-Thoracic Surgery (EACTS). European Heart Journal. 2015;**36**(42):2921-2964

[3] Imazio M, Adler Y. Management of pericardial effusion. European Heart Journal. 2013;**34**(16):1186-1197

[4] Shabetai R. Pericardial effusion: haemodynamic spectrum. Heart. 2004;**90**(3):255-256

[5] Sagrista-Sauleda J, Merce J, Permanyer-Miralda G, Soler-Soler J. Clinical clues to the causes of large pericardial effusions. The American Journal of Medicine. 2000;**109**(2):95-101

[6] Merce J, Sagrista Sauleda J, Permanyer Miralda G, Carballo J, Olona M, Soler Soler J. Pericardial effusion in the elderly: A different disease? Revista Española de Cardiología. 2000;**53**(11):1432-1436

[7] Sagrista-Sauleda J, Merce AS, Soler-Soler J. Diagnosis and management of pericardial effusion. World Journal of Cardiology. 2011;**3**(5):135-143

[8] Khandaker MH, Espinosa RE, Nishimura RA, Sinak LJ, Hayes SN, Melduni RM, et al. Pericardial disease: Diagnosis and management. Mayo Clinic Proceedings. 2010;**85**(6):572-593

[9] Sarkar M, Bhardwaj R, Madabhavi I, Gowda S, Dogra K. Pulsus paradoxus. The Clinical Respiratory Journal. 2018;**12**(8):2321-2331

[10] Imazio M, Spodick DH, Brucato A, Trinchero R, Adler Y. Controversial issues in the management of pericardial diseases. Circulation. 2010;**121**(7):916-928

[11] Yared K, Baggish AL, Picard MH, Hoffmann U, Hung J. Multimodality imaging of pericardial diseases. JACC: Cardiovascular Imaging. 2010;**3**(6):650-660

[12] De Filippo O, Gatti P, Rettegno S, Iannaccone M, D'Ascenzo F, Lazaros G, et al. Is pericardial effusion a negative prognostic marker? Meta-analysis of outcomes of pericardial effusion. Journal of Cardiovascular Medicine. 2019;**20**(1):39-45

[13] Spodick D. The Pericardium, a Comprehensive Textbook. New York: Marcel Dekker; 1997. p. 260

[14] Spodick D. Pericardial disease. In: Braunwald E, Zipes D, Libby P, editors. Heart Disease: A Textbook of Cardiovascular Medicine. New York: Saunders; 2001. p. 183

[15] Imazio M, Gaita F, LeWinter M. Evaluation and treatment of pericarditis: A systematic review. Journal of the American Medical Association. 2015;**314**(14):1498-1506

[16] Heidenreich PA, Eisenberg MJ, Kee LL, Somelofski CA, Hollander H, Schiller NB, et al. Pericardial effusion in AIDS. Incidence and survival. Circulation. 1995;**92**(11):3229-3234

[17] Chen Y, Brennessel D, Walters J, Johnson M, Rosner F, Raza M. Human

immunodeficiency virus-associated pericardial effusion: Report of 40 cases and review of the literature. American Heart Journal. 1999;**137**(3):516-521

[18] Levy PY, Corey R, Berger P, Habib G, Bonnet JL, Levy S, et al. Etiologic diagnosis of 204 pericardial effusions. Medicine. 2003;**82**(6):385-391

[19] Permanyer-Miralda G, Sagrista-Sauleda J, Soler-Soler J. Primary acute pericardial disease: A prospective series of 231 consecutive patients. The American Journal of Cardiology. 1985;**56**(10):623-630

[20] Zayas R, Anguita M, Torres F, Gimenez D, Bergillos F, Ruiz M, et al. Incidence of specific etiology and role of methods for specific etiologic diagnosis of primary acute pericarditis. The American Journal of Cardiology. 1995;**75**(5):378-382

[21] Galve E, Garcia-Del-Castillo H, Evangelista A, Batlle J, Permanyer-Miralda G, Soler-Soler J. Pericardial effusion in the course of myocardial infarction: Incidence, natural history, and clinical relevance. Circulation. 1986;**73**(2):294-299

[22] Correale E, Maggioni AP, Romano S, Ricciardiello V, Battista R, Salvarola G, et al. Comparison of frequency, diagnostic and prognostic significance of pericardial involvement in acute myocardial infarction treated with and without thrombolytics. Gruppo Italiano per lo studio della Sopravvivenza nell'Infarto Miocardico (GISSI). The American Journal of Cardiology. 1993;**71**(16):1377-1381

[23] Belkin RN, Mark DB, Aronson L, Szwed H, Califf RM, Kisslo J. Pericardial effusion after intravenous recombinant tissue-type plasminogen activator for acute myocardial infarction. The American Journal of Cardiology. 1991;**67**(6):496-500

[24] Shahar A, Hod H, Barabash GM, Kaplinsky E, Motro M. Disappearance of a syndrome: Dressler's syndrome in the era of thrombolysis. Cardiology. 1994;**85**(3-4):255-258

[25] Stewart JR, Fajardo LF, Gillette SM, Constine LS. Radiation injury to the heart. International Journal of Radiation Oncology, Biology, Physics. 1995;**31**(5):1205-1211

[26] Rostand SG, Rutsky EA. Pericarditis in end-stage renal disease. Cardiology Clinics. 1990;**8**(4):701-707

[27] Gunukula SR, Spodick DH. Pericardial disease in renal patients. Seminars in Nephrology. 2001;**21**(1):52-56

[28] Kabadi UM, Kumar SP. Pericardial effusion in primary hypothyroidism. American Heart Journal. 1990;**120** (6 Pt 1):1393-1395

[29] Imazio M. Myopericardial Diseases. New York: Springer; 2016

[30] Spodick DH. Acute pericarditis: Current concepts and practice. Journal of the American Medical Association. 2003;**289**(9):1150-1153

[31] Troughton RW, Asher CR, Klein AL. Pericarditis. Lancet. 2004;**363**(9410):717-727

[32] Imazio M, Demichelis B, Parrini I, Giuggia M, Cecchi E, Gaschino G, et al. Day-hospital treatment of acute pericarditis: A management program for outpatient therapy. Journal of the American College of Cardiology. 2004;**43**(6):1042-1046

[33] Imazio M, Cecchi E, Demichelis B, Ierna S, Demarie D, Ghisio A, et al. Indicators of poor prognosis of acute pericarditis. Circulation. 2007;**115**(21): 2739-2744

[34] Imazio M, Demichelis B, Cecchi E, Belli R, Ghisio A, Bobbio M, et al. Cardiac

troponin I in acute pericarditis. Journal of the American College of Cardiology. 2003;**42**(12):2144-2148

[35] Klein AL, Abbara S, Agler DA, Appleton CP, Asher CR, Hoit B, et al. American Society of Echocardiography clinical recommendations for multimodality cardiovascular imaging of patients with pericardial disease: Endorsed by the Society for Cardiovascular Magnetic Resonance and Society of cardiovascular computed tomography. Journal of the American Society of Echocardiography. 2013;**26**(9):965-1012.e15

[36] Rutsky EA, Rostand SG. Pericarditis in end-stage renal disease: Clinical characteristics and management. Seminars in Dialysis. 1989;**2**(1):25-30

[37] Spodick DH. Arrhythmias during acute pericarditis. A prospective study of 100 consecutive cases. Journal of the American Medical Association. 1976;**235**(1):39-41

[38] Imazio M, Cecchi E, Demichelis B, Chinaglia A, Ierna S, Demarie D, et al. Myopericarditis versus viral or idiopathic acute pericarditis. Heart. 2008;**94**(4):498-501

[39] Imazio M, Bobbio M, Cecchi E, Demarie D, Demichelis B, Pomari F, et al. Colchicine in addition to conventional therapy for acute pericarditis: Results of the COlchicine for acute PEricarditis (COPE) trial. Circulation. 2005;**112**(13):2012-2016

[40] Hammerman H, Alker KJ, Schoen FJ, Kloner RA. Morphologic and functional effects of piroxicam on myocardial scar formation after coronary occlusion in dogs. The American Journal of Cardiology. 1984;**53**(4):604-607

[41] Imazio M, Brucato A, Maestroni S, Cumetti D, Dominelli A, Natale G, et al. Prevalence of C-reactive protein elevation and time course of normalization in acute pericarditis: Implications for the diagnosis, therapy, and prognosis of pericarditis. Circulation. 2011;**123**(10):1092-1097

[42] Imazio M, Cecchi E, Ierna S, Trinchero R, ICAP Investigators. Investigation on colchicine for acute pericarditis: A multicenter randomized placebo-controlled trial evaluating the clinical benefits of colchicine as adjunct to conventional therapy in the treatment and prevention of pericarditis; study design amd rationale. Journal of Cardiovascular Medicine. 2007;**8**(8):613-617

[43] Alabed S, Cabello JB, Irving GJ, Qintar M, Burls A. Colchicine for pericarditis. Cochrane Database of Systematic Reviews. 2014;**8**:CD010652. DOI: 10.1002/14651858.CD010652.pub2

[44] Lotrionte M, Biondi-Zoccai G, Imazio M, Castagno D, Moretti C, Abbate A, et al. International collaborative systematic review of controlled clinical trials on pharmacologic treatments for acute pericarditis and its recurrences. American Heart Journal. 2010;**160**(4):662-670

[45] Mody P, Bikdeli B, Wang Y, Imazio M, Krumholz HM. Trends in acute pericarditis hospitalizations and outcomes among the elderly in the USA, 1999-2012. European Heart Journal—Quality of Care and Clinical Outcomes. 2018;**4**(2):98-105

[46] Robinson J, Brigden W. Recurrent pericarditis. British Medical Journal. 1968;**2**(5600):272-275

[47] Fowler NO. Recurrent pericarditis. Cardiology Clinics. 1990;**8**(4):621-626

[48] Fowler NO, Harbin AD 3rd. Recurrent acute pericarditis: Follow-up study of 31 patients. Journal of the

American College of Cardiology. 1986;**7**(2):300-305

[49] Maisch B, Ristic AD, Pankuweit S. Intrapericardial treatment of autoreactive pericardial effusion with triamcinolone; the way to avoid side effects of systemic corticosteroid therapy. European Heart Journal. 2002;**23**(19):1503-1508

[50] Pankuweit S, Wadlich A, Meyer E, Portig I, Hufnagel G, Maisch B. Cytokine activation in pericardial fluids in different forms of pericarditis. Herz. 2000;**25**(8):748-754

[51] Brucato A, Brambilla G, Moreo A, Alberti A, Munforti C, Ghirardello A, et al. Long-term outcomes in difficult-to-treat patients with recurrent pericarditis. The American Journal of Cardiology. 2006;**98**(2):267-271

[52] Imazio M, Bobbio M, Cecchi E, Demarie D, Pomari F, Moratti M, et al. Colchicine as first-choice therapy for recurrent pericarditis: Results of the CORE (COlchicine for REcurrent pericarditis) trial. Archives of Internal Medicine. 2005;**165**(17):1987-1991

[53] Soler-Soler J, Sagrista-Sauleda J, Permanyer-Miralda G. Relapsing pericarditis. Heart. 2004;**90**(11): 1364-1368

[54] Imazio M, Demichelis B, Parrini I, Cecchi E, Demarie D, Ghisio A, et al. Management, risk factors, and outcomes in recurrent pericarditis. The American Journal of Cardiology. 2005;**96**(5):736-739

[55] Lange RA, Hillis LD. Clinical practice. Acute pericarditis. The New England Journal of Medicine. 2004;**351**(21):2195-2202

[56] Artom G, Koren-Morag N, Spodick DH, Brucato A, Guindo J, Bayes-de-Luna A, et al. Pretreatment with corticosteroids attenuates the efficacy of colchicine in preventing recurrent pericarditis: A multi-centre all-case analysis. European Heart Journal. 2005;**26**(7):723-727

[57] Imazio M, Brucato A, Mayosi BM, Derosa FG, Lestuzzi C, Macor A, et al. Medical therapy of pericardial diseases: Part I: Idiopathic and infectious pericarditis. Journal of Cardiovascular Medicine. 2010;**11**(10):712-722

[58] Markel G, Imazio M, Brucato A, Adler Y. Prevention of recurrent pericarditis with colchicine in 2012. Clinical Cardiology. 2013;**36**(3):125-128

[59] Brucato A, Imazio M, Gattorno M, Lazaros G, Maestroni S, Carraro M, et al. Effect of anakinra on recurrent pericarditis among patients with colchicine resistance and corticosteroid dependence: The AIRTRIP randomized clinical trial. Journal of the American Medical Association. 2016;**316**(18):1906-1912

[60] LeWinter M, Imazio M. Pericardial disease. In: Braunwald E, Zipes D, Libby P, editors. Heart Disease: A Textbook of Cardiovascular Medicine. New York: Saunders; 2018

[61] Cosyns B, Plein S, Nihoyanopoulos P, Smiseth O, Achenbach S, Andrade MJ, et al. European Association of Cardiovascular Imaging (EACVI) position paper: Multimodality imaging in pericardial disease. European Heart Journal Cardiovascular Imaging. 2015;**16**(1):12-31

[62] Imazio M, Pedrotti P, Quattrocchi G, Roghi A, Badano L, Faletti R, et al. Multimodality imaging of pericardial diseases. Journal of Cardiovascular Medicine. 2016;**17**(11):774-782

[63] Welch TD. Constrictive pericarditis: Diagnosis, management and clinical outcomes. Heart. 2018;**104**(9):725-731

[64] Cameron J, Oesterle SN, Baldwin JC, Hancock EW. The etiologic spectrum of constrictive pericarditis. American Heart Journal. 1987;**113** (2 Pt 1):354-360

[65] Ling LH, Oh JK, Schaff HV, Danielson GK, Mahoney DW, Seward JB, et al. Constrictive pericarditis in the modern era: Evolving clinical spectrum and impact on outcome after pericardiectomy. Circulation. 1999;**100**(13):1380-1386

[66] Bertog SC, Thambidorai SK, Parakh K, Schoenhagen P, Ozduran V, Houghtaling PL, et al. Constrictive pericarditis: Etiology and cause-specific survival after pericardiectomy. Journal of the American College of Cardiology. 2004;**43**(8):1445-1452

[67] Szabo G, Schmack B, Bulut C, Soos P, Weymann A, Stadtfeld S, et al. Constrictive pericarditis: Risks, aetiologies and outcomes after total pericardiectomy: 24 years of experience. European Journal of Cardio-Thoracic Surgery. 2013;**44**(6):1023-1028; discussion 1028

[68] George TJ, Arnaoutakis GJ, Beaty CA, Kilic A, Baumgartner WA, Conte JV. Contemporary etiologies, risk factors, and outcomes after pericardiectomy. The Annals of Thoracic Surgery. 2012;**94**(2):445-451

[69] Vistarini N, Chen C, Mazine A, Bouchard D, Hebert Y, Carrier M, et al. Pericardiectomy for constrictive pericarditis: 20 years of experience at the Montreal heart institute. The Annals of Thoracic Surgery. 2015;**100**(1):107-113

[70] Mutyaba AK, Balkaran S, Cloete R, du Plessis N, Badri M, Brink J, et al. Constrictive pericarditis requiring pericardiectomy at Groote Schuur hospital, Cape Town, South Africa: Causes and perioperative outcomes in the HIV era (1990-2012). The Journal of Thoracic and Cardiovascular Surgery. 2014;**148**(6):3058-65.e1

[71] Spodick DH. The normal and diseased pericardium: Current concepts of pericardial physiology, diagnosis and treatment. Journal of the American College of Cardiology. 1983;**1**(1):240-251

[72] Welch TD, Ling LH, Espinosa RE, Anavekar NS, Wiste HJ, Lahr BD, et al. Echocardiographic diagnosis of constrictive pericarditis: Mayo Clinic criteria. Circulation. Cardiovascular Imaging. 2014;**7**(3):526-534

[73] Cheitlin MD, Armstrong WF, Aurigemma GP, Beller GA, Bierman FZ, Davis JL, et al. ACC/AHA/ASE 2003 guideline update for the clinical application of echocardiography: Summary article: A report of the American College of Cardiology/ American Heart Association task force on practice guidelines (ACC/AHA/ ASE Committee to update the 1997 guidelines for the clinical application of echocardiography). Circulation. 2003;**108**(9):1146-1162

[74] Talreja DR, Nishimura RA, Oh JK, Holmes DR. Constrictive pericarditis in the modern era: Novel criteria for diagnosis in the cardiac catheterization laboratory. Journal of the American College of Cardiology. 2008;**51**(3):315-319

[75] Verhaert D, Gabriel RS, Johnston D, Lytle BW, Desai MY, Klein AL. The role of multimodality imaging in the management of pericardial disease. Circulation. Cardiovascular Imaging. 2010;**3**(3):333-343

[76] Chang SA, Choi JY, Kim EK, Hyun SH, Jang SY, Choi JO, et al. [^{18}F]Fluorodeoxyglucose PET/CT predicts response to steroid therapy in constrictive pericarditis. Journal of the American College of Cardiology. 2017;**69**(6):750-752

[77] Spodick DH. Acute cardiac tamponade. The New England Journal of Medicine. 2003;**349**(7):684-690

[78] Adlam DFJ. Pericardial disease. Medicine. 2018;**46**(11):703-708

[79] Restrepo CS, Lemos DF, Lemos JA, Velasquez E, Diethelm L, Ovella TA, et al. Imaging findings in cardiac tamponade with emphasis on CT. Radiographics. 2007;**27**(6):1595-1610

[80] Ristic AD, Imazio M, Adler Y, Anastasakis A, Badano LP, Brucato A, et al. Triage strategy for urgent management of cardiac tamponade: A position statement of the European Society of Cardiology Working Group on myocardial and pericardial diseases. European Heart Journal. 2014;**35**(34):2279-2284

Chapter 3

Tuberculous Pericarditis

Picco José Miguel

Abstract

The pericardium formed by two layers, pleural and visceral, fulfills the role of keeping the heart in position and in turn acts as a barrier against infections. Their commitment may be due to a wide variety of rare diseases where the causes are usually idiopathic, inflammatory, neoplastic, traumatic, congenital, or infectious. Within the latter they are of viral, fungal, and bacterial origin, being able to be caused by *Mycobacteria*. Tuberculous pericarditis is the entity in which inflammation of the pericardium is caused by Koch's bacillus. The access route to it includes three mechanisms: (1) lymphatic; (2) hematogenous spread, mainly in immunocompetent patients; and (3) by direct contact from adjacent structures such as the lung and pleura. In immunocompetent patients, the condition is usually paucibacillary, with manifestation at the level of a single organ, while in immunocompromised patients, the rate of bacterial replication is high. Tuberculosis (TB) is a disease that is far from being eradicated today. Despite the great majority of cases in which pulmonary involvement is confirmed, a large number of patients suffer compromises from other organs. If tuberculous pericarditis is suspected, it is important to be able to establish an early diagnosis in order to achieve an adequate treatment as soon as possible.

Keywords: pericarditis, pericardium, tuberculosis, infection

1. Introduction

Tuberculosis (TB) has decreased its incidence in the industrialized countries in the last 100 years; despite this it remains within the top 10 of infectious diseases that cause death (above HIV). Millions of people contract TB every year [1]. Tuberculous pericarditis, caused by *Mycobacterium tuberculosis* (Mtb), is a rare disease, observed in about 2% of people suffering from pulmonary tuberculosis and about 1% in autopsies of people who die from tuberculosis [2].

2. Epidemiology

According to the global report of TB 2018, it is estimated that about 10 million people developed the disease during 2017. Cases were reported in all countries and age groups, but the majority (90%) occurred in adults (>15 years old). Nearly 9% of infected people were HIV carriers (72% in Africa). Two thirds of the cases were reported in eight countries: India (27%), China (9%), Indonesia (8%), the Philippines (6%), Pakistan (5%), Nigeria (4%), Bangladesh (4%), and South Africa (3%). Only 6% of the cases were reported in the European region and 3% in the region of the Americas [1].

3. Pathogenesis of tuberculous pericarditis

Tubercle bacilli access the pericardium via three mechanisms: (1) retrograde lymphatic spread from mediastinal, paratracheal, and peribronchial lymph nodes [3], (2) hematogenous spread (dominant in immunocompromised hosts) [4], and (3) direct contiguous spread from adjacent structures such as the lungs, pleura, and spine (infrequent) [3]. When the guest is immunocompetent, tuberculous pericardial disease is localized to the pericardial space. Usually in a paucibacillary condition, tubercle proteins trigger an important cell-mediated hypersensitivity response with T-helper cell (subtype 1) predominant cytokine release, leading to an inflammatory exudative effusion and its hemodynamic sequelae [5, 6]. The immune response to the viable acid-fast bacilli penetrating the pericardium is responsible for the morbidity associated with tuberculous pericarditis. In patients with dysfunctional immunity as occurred in HIV/AIDS, there is evidence that mycobacterial replication is active, bacillary loads are high, and the clinical manifestations of tuberculous pericarditis are related to the impact of the infectious and virulent nature of the Mtb itself in addition to the hemodynamic sequelae [4–7].

There are four pathological stages of tuberculous pericarditis: (1) fibrinous exudation, initial polymorphonuclear leukocytosis, abundant mycobacteria, and early granuloma formation with loose organization of macrophages and T cells; (2) serosanguineous effusion with a predominantly lymphocytic exudate with monocytes and foam cells; (3) absorption of effusion with organization of granulomatous caseation and pericardial thickening caused by fibrin, collagenosis, and, ultimately, fibrosis; and (4) constrictive scarring. The fibrosis generated between the visceral pericardium and the parietal pericardium can calcify and adhere to the myocardium, generating a cuirass around the heart, preventing the correct diastolic filling, and generating the clinical syndrome of constrictive pericarditis [8].

Tuberculous pericarditis presents clinically in three forms: pericardial effusion, constrictive pericarditis, and a combination of effusion and constriction.

4. Pericardial effusion

The triad of severe pericarditic chest pain: a pericardial friction rub, widespread ST segment, and T-wave abnormalities; and PR segment depression typical of acute pericarditis is an uncommon clinical presentation of tuberculous pericarditis, accounting for only 3–8% of patients who present with tuberculous pericarditis [9]. The pericardial effusion begins as soon as the tubercle bacillus enters the pericardium and develops slowly and insidiously. Is characterized pathologically by polymorphonuclear leukocytosis with abundant bacilli and granuloma formation, and is usually present with nonspecific systemic symptoms, such as fever, night sweats, fatigue, and weight loss. Chest pain, cough, and breathlessness are uncommon symptoms [10].

TB pericarditis should be considered in the evaluation of all cases of pericarditis without a rapidly self-limited course.

4.1 Diagnosis of pericardial effusion

ECG is abnormal in most cases of tuberculous pericardial effusion, usually in the form of nonspecific ST-T-wave changes. The presence of microvoltage (complexes <5 mm in limb leads and <10 mm in precordial leads) suggests a large pericardial effusion [11]. Chest radiograph usually shows an enlarged cardiac shadow in more than 90% of cases and demonstrates features of active pulmonary TB in 30% of cases and pleural effusion in 40–60% of cases (**Figure 1**) [12]. The advent and accessibility of echocardiography have made it possible to diagnose the pericardial effusion when suspected; however, it does not determine the etiology. The presence of fibrinous strands on the visceral pericardium is typical but not specific for a tuberculous pathogenesis (Video 1, https://bit.ly/2JNuQdB) [13]. Computed tomography of the chest shows typical changes in mediastinal lymph nodes (enlargement >10 mm with matting and hypodense centers and sparing of hilar lymph nodes) in almost 100% of cases [14].

4.2 Direct methods for the diagnosis of tuberculous pericarditis

The pericardial fluid is bloodstained in 80% of cases of tuberculous pericarditis, but malignant disease and the late effects of penetrating trauma may also cause bloody pericardial effusion, so confirmation of TB as the cause is important [15]. Tuberculous pericardial effusions are typically exudative and characterized by a high protein content and increased leukocyte count, with a predominance of lymphocytes and monocytes. Light's criteria (whereby an exudate is defined as having one or more of the following: pleural fluid protein divided by serum protein >0.5, pleural fluid lactate dehydrogenase [LDH] divided by serum LDH >0.6, and/or pleural fluid LDH level > 66% of the upper limit of normal for serum LDH) [16] is the most reliable diagnostic tool for identifying pericardial exudates.

The definitive diagnosis of tuberculous pericarditis should be established as soon as possible, by searching for the acid-alcohol bacilli resistant in sputum, lymph nodes, or pericardial fluid [17]. Culture of tubercle bacilli from pericardial fluid can be improved by inoculation of the fluid into double-strength liquid Kirchner

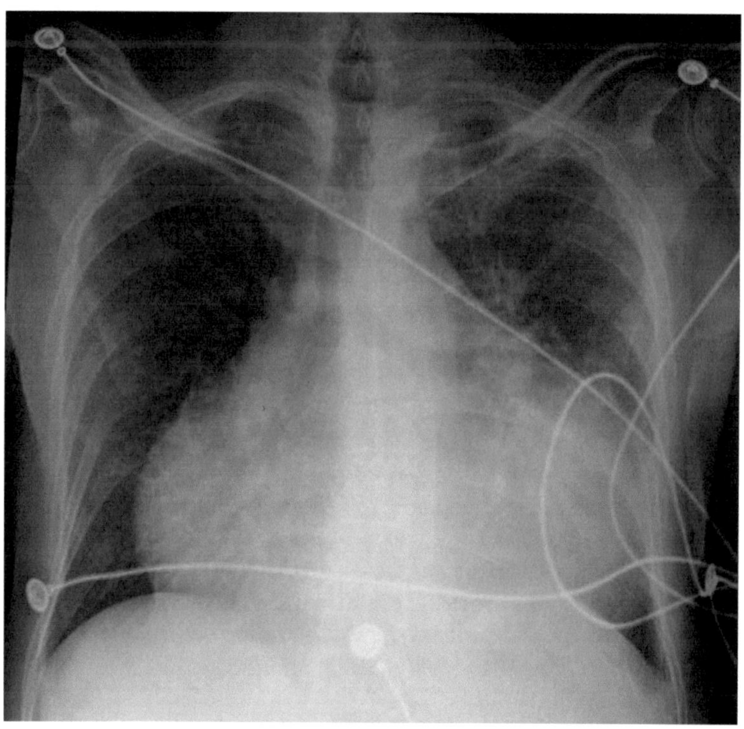

Figure 1.
Chest X-ray in front of a merchant marine patient who consulted due to progressive dyspnea for months of evolution. In the consultation, he presented signs of cardiac tamponade, so an echocardiogram (Video 1, https://bit.ly/2JNuQdB) was performed with an evacuating pericardiocentesis of 3 liters of hematopurulent fluid. Bacteriological isolation was not obtained, but there was increased ADA activity.

culture medium, resulting in a 75% yield, compared with a 53% yield with conventional culture [18]. Pericardial biopsy specimens may also be used to diagnose tuberculous pericarditis. The polymerase chain reaction (PCR) has also been suggested for detecting *M. tuberculosis* DNA in pericardial fluid [19]. The probability of obtaining a definitive bacteriological result is greatest when pericardial fluid and biopsy specimens are examined early in the effusive stage [18].

4.3 Indirect methods for the diagnosis of tuberculous pericarditis

The difficulty of carrying out the diagnosis of tuberculous pericarditis, associated with its high mortality without proper treatment, has led to the use of indirect methods. Indirect methods such as dosing activity of adenosine deaminase (ADA) in the pericardial fluid, with cut-off levels between 30 and 60 U/L of ADA activity, are suggestive of tuberculous pericarditis [20]. In areas of the high endemic level of tuberculosis, a cut-off level of ADA activity <35 presents a sensitivity of 90% and a specificity of 74% for diagnosis [21]. The utility of ADA activity in pericardial fluid was also demonstrated in HIV-positive patients, although in patients with severe CD4 lymphocyte depletion, the ADA levels observed are lower [22].

Very high levels of ADA in pericardial fluid have strong association with constrictive pericarditis [23].

The measurement of interferon gamma (IFN-γ) levels in the pericardial fluid also helps early diagnosis. Cut-off values >200 pg/L have a sensitivity of 92% and specificity of 100% for the diagnosis of TB [21].

In summary, the "definitive" diagnosis of tuberculous pericarditis is based on the presence of the tubercle bacillus in the pericardial fluid or proving it in the pericardium biopsy and "probably" when there is evidence of tuberculosis elsewhere in the body and the presence of unexplained pericarditis, with high levels of ADA or good response to pharmacological treatment.

5. Treatment

Pharmacological treatment increases survival in tuberculous pericarditis, even in HIV-positive patients [24]. A regimen that includes rifampicin, isoniazid, pyrazinamide, and ethambutol for at least 2 months, followed by rifampicin and isoniazid (up to 6 months), proved to be effective in extrapulmonary tuberculosis [25]. Treatments beyond 6 months do not show better results, increasing cost and decreasing tolerance [26].

The treatment associated with corticosteroids would not be justified at present, given that the evidence for its use is not the best [27]. Although the results are inconclusive, adding corticosteroids to treatment may have benefits on morbidity and re-experiences, but randomized controlled trials with sufficient numbers of HIV-positive and HIV-negative patients are needed [28].

It is obvious that if pericarditis is associated with severe pericardial effusion, with hemodynamic compromise, the first treatment option associated with antituberculous treatment is drainage by subxiphoid puncture or by minimal thoracotomy.

6. Constrictive pericarditis

It is the most feared complication of tuberculous pericarditis; it is described in about 30% of patients, even in spite of antituberculous treatment and the use of corticosteroids [29]. The clinical presentation can be variable, from asymptomatic patients and stress design to heart failure with preserved function, liver failure (due to retrograde passive congestion) with ascites, and generalized edema. The presence of pericardial knock, associated with protodiastolic murmur, splitting of the second heart sound, and Kussmaul's sign (paradoxical increase in jugular venous pressure in inspiration), is frequent in constrictive pericarditis but difficult to detect by non-experienced observers [30].

6.1 Diagnosis of constrictive pericarditis

Sometimes we can see a calcium shell surrounding the heart in the chest X-ray, but it is not the most frequent [31]. Other nonspecific radiographic findings are dilation of the superior vena cava [12].

In the electrocardiogram there are no specific signs, either atrial fibrillation, nonspecific alterations of repolarization (changes in the T wave), or complexes with low voltage.

The Doppler echocardiogram may show thickening of the pericardium; the presence of fibrin; restrictive transmitral filling pattern, associated with normal size of the cavities, in the absence of ventricular hypertrophy; and valvular insufficiency.

6.2 Treatment

The treatment must include antituberculous medication for 6 months. Consider pericardiectomy in all patients once antibiotic treatment has been instituted [32]. Surgery should be performed early if the patient presents hemodynamic deterioration (despite antituberculous treatment) [33] or if they present pericardial calcifications, which are markers of chronicity of the disease [34].

7. Effusive constrictive pericarditis

It is the presence of increased intrapericardial pressure due to effusion and constriction of the visceral pericardium, which does not improve with pericardiocentesis. The signs and symptoms are similar to those of constrictive pericarditis.

The treatment is pericardiectomy associated with antituberculous treatment for 6 months.

8. Conclusions

Tuberculous pericarditis is a rare pathology in developed countries but frequent in developing countries. There is difficulty in the diagnosis due to low bacteriological and histological results. The usefulness of indirect methods for diagnosis should be taken into account, especially in patients with torpid pericarditis. The presence of positive serology for HIV can modify the clinical presentation and the outcome of tuberculous pericarditis.

There is still a lack of sustainable evidence for the use of systemic corticosteroids in this pathology.

Pharmacological treatment should be performed for at least 6 months in all patients with tuberculous pericarditis, regardless of drainage or pericardiectomy.

Author details

Picco José Miguel
Wolff Institute of Sports and Cardiology/Doppler Echocardiography Service—Italian Hospital, Mendoza City, Argentina

*Address all correspondence to: piccojose@gmail.com

IntechOpen

© 2019 The Author(s). Licensee IntechOpen. This chapter is distributed under the terms of the Creative Commons Attribution License (http://creativecommons.org/licenses/by/3.0), which permits unrestricted use, distribution, and reproduction in any medium, provided the original work is properly cited.

References

[1] World Health Organization. Global Tuberculosis Report 2018. Available from: https://www.who.int/tb/publications/global_report/en/. ISBN 978-92-4-156564-6 2018

[2] Fowler NO. Tuberculous pericarditis. Journal of the American Medical Association. 1991;**266**:99-103

[3] Spodick DH. Tuberculous pericarditis. A.M.A. Archives of Internal Medicine. 1956;**98**(6):737-749

[4] Ntsekhe M, Mayosi BM. Tuberculous pericarditis with and without HIV. Heart Failure Reviews. 2013;**18**(3):367-373

[5] Mayosi BM, Burgess LJ, Doubell AF. Tuberculous pericarditis. Circulation. 2005;**112**(23):3608-3616

[6] Burgess LJ, Reuter H, Taljaard JJF, Doubell AF. Role of biochemical tests in the diagnosis of large pericardial effusions. Chest. 2002;**121**:495-499

[7] Pasipanodya JG, Mubanga M, Ntsekhe M, Pandie S, Magazi BT, Gumedze F, et al. Tuberculous pericarditis is multibacillary and bacterial burden drives high mortality. eBioMedicine. 2015;**2**(11):1634-1639

[8] Tirilomis T, Univerdorben S, von der Emde J. Pericardectomy for chronic constrictive pericarditis: Risks and outcome. European Journal of Cardio-Thoracic Surgery. 1994;**8**:487-492

[9] Mayosi BM, Wiysonge CS, Ntsekhe M, Volmink JA, Gumedze F, Maartens G, et al. Clinical characteristics and initial management of patients with tuberculous pericarditis in the HIV era: The investigation of the management of pericarditis in Africa (IMPI Africa) registry. BMC Infectious Diseases. 2006;**6**(2)

[10] Schrire V. Experience with pericarditis at Groote Schuur Hospital, Cape Town: An analysis of one hundred and sixty cases over a six-year period. South African Medical Journal. 1959;**33**:810-817

[11] Smedema JP, Katjitae I, Reuter H, Burgess L, Louw V, Pretorius M, et al. Twelve-lead electrocardiography in tuberculous pericarditis. Cardiovascular Journal of South Africa. 2001;**12**:31-34

[12] Reuter H, Burgess LJ, Doubell AF. The role of chest radiography in diagnosing patients with tuberculous pericarditis. Cardiovascular Journal of Southern Africa. 2005;**16**:108-111

[13] Liu PY, Li YH, Tsai WC, Chao TH, Yung YJ, Chen JH. Usefulness of echocardiographic intrapericardial abnormalities in the diagnosis of tuberculous pericardial effusion. The American Journal of Cardiology. 2001;**87**:1133-1135

[14] Cherian G. Diagnosis of tuberculous aetiology in pericardial effusions. Postgraduate Medical Journal 2004;**80**:262-266

[15] Mayosi BM, Volmink JA, Commerford PJ. Pericardial disease: An evidence-based approach to diagnosis and treatment. In: Yusuf S, Cairns JA, Camm AJ, Fallen BJ, editors. Evidence-Based Cardiology. 2nd ed. London: BMJ Books; 2003. pp. 735-748

[16] Burgess LJ, Reuter H, Carstens ME, Taljaard JJ, Doubell AF. Cytokine production in patients with tuberculous pericarditis. The International Journal of Tuberculosis and Lung Disease. 2002;**6**:439-446

[17] Hageman JH, d'Esopo ND, Glenn WWL. Tuberculosis of the pericardium:

A long-term analysis of forty-four proved cases. The New England Journal of Medicine. 1964;**270**:327-332

[18] Strang G, Latouf S, Commerford P, Roditi D, Duncan-Traill G, Barlow D, et al. Bedside culture to confirm tuberculous pericarditis. Lancet. 1991;**338**:1600-1601

[19] Cegielski JP, Devlin BH, Morris AJ, Kitinya JN, Pulipaka UP, Lema LEK, et al. Comparison of PCR, culture and histopathology for the diagnosis of tuberculous pericarditis. Journal of Clinical Microbiology. 1997;**35**:3254-3257

[20] Martinez-Vasquez JM, Ribera E, Ocana I, Segura RM, Serrat R, Sagrista J. Adenosine deaminase activity in tuberculous pericarditis. Thorax. 1986;**41**:888-889

[21] Burgess LJ, Reuter H, Carstens ME, Taljaard JJF, Doubell AF. The use of adenosine deaminase and interferon-gamma as diagnostic tools for tuberculous pericarditis. Chest. 2002;**122**:900-905

[22] Reuter H, Burgess LJ, Carstens ME, Doubell AF. Adenosine deaminase activity: More than a diagnostic tool in tuberculous pericarditis. Cardiovascular Journal of Southern Africa. 2005;**16**:143-147

[23] Komsouglu B, Goldeli O, Kulan K, Komsouglu SS. The diagnostic and prognostic value of adenosine deaminase in tuberculous pericarditis. European Heart Journal. 1995;**16**:1126-1130

[24] Hakim JG, Ternouth I, Mushangi E, Siziya S, Robertson V, Malin A. Double blind randomised placebo controlled trial of adjunctive prednisolone in the treatment of effusive tuberculous pericarditis in HIV seropositive patients. Heart. 2000;**84**:183-188

[25] Cohn DL, Catlin BJ, Peterson KL, Judson FN, Sbarbaro JA. A 62-dose, 6-month therapy for pulmonary and extrapulmonary tuberculosis: A twice-weekly directly-observed, cost-effective regimen. Annals of Internal Medicine. 1990;**112**:407-415

[26] Combs DL, O'Brien RJ, Geiter LJ. USPHS Tuberculosis Short-Course Chemotherapy Trial 21: Effectiveness, toxicity and acceptability: The report of final results. Annals of Internal Medicine. 1990;**112**:397-406

[27] Freers J, Hakim J, Myanja-Kizza H, Parry E. The heart. In: Parry E, Godfrey R, Mabey D, Gill G, editors. Principles of Medicine in Africa. 3rd ed. Cambridge, UK: Cambridge University Press; 2004. pp. 837-886

[28] Ntsekhe M, Wiysonge C, Volmink JA, Commerford PJ, Mayosi BM. Adjuvant corticosteroids for tuberculous pericarditis: Promising, but not proven. The Quarterly Journal of Medicine. 2003;**96**:593-599

[29] Sagrista-Sauleda J, Permanyer-Miralda G, Soler-Soler J. Tuberculous pericarditis: Ten-year experience with a prospective protocol for diagnosis and treatment. Journal of the American College of Cardiology. 1988;**11**:724-728

[30] Commerford PJ, Strang JIG. Tuberculous pericarditis. In: Coovadia HM, Benatar SR, editors. A Century of Tuberculosis: South African Perspectives. Cape Town: Oxford University Press; 1991. pp. 123-136

[31] Strang JIG, Kakaza HHS, Gibson DG, Allen BW, Mitchison DA, Evans DJ, et al. Controlled trial of prednisolone as adjuvant in treatment of tuberculous constrictive pericarditis in Transkei. Lancet. 1987;**2**:1418-1422

[32] Sonneberg FA, Parker SG. Elective pericardiectomy for tuberculous

pericarditis. Medical Decision Making. 1986;**6**:110-123

[33] Long R, Younes M, Patton N, Hershfield E. Tuberculous pericarditis: Long-term outcome in patients who received medical therapy alone. American Heart Journal. 1989;**117**:1133-1139

[34] Bashi VV, John S, Ravikumar E, Jairaj PS, Shyamsunder K, Krishnaswami S. Early and late results of pericardiectomy in 118 cases of constrictive pericarditis. Thorax. 1988;**43**:637-641

Chapter 4

Chronic Constrictive Pericarditis (CCP) in Africa: Epidemiology, Etiology, Diagnosis, and Surgical Treatment

Koffi Herve Yangni-Angate

"What has been accomplished does not die, but too often alas, the personality of those who have handed the torch from one generation to another soon fades into oblivion."
Harvey Cushing (as quoted in Harvey Cushing: A Biography by John F. Fulton, 1947)

Abstract

Chronic constrictive pericarditis (CCP) is not rare in Africa with tuberculosis as the most common etiology. A long history of visceral tuberculosis, typical symptoms of CCP because of late clinical presentation in most cases, make diagnosis almost easy to establish. Echocardiography and cardiac catheterization may be helpful as final investigation when differentiation between CCP, endomyocardial fibrosis, and restrictive ventricular heart disease is difficult to attest. Pericardiectomy remains the only efficient treatment to carry out. We review the African teams' surgical experiences on pericardiectomy and report their surgical results and those worldwide in literature overall. In African groups, early mortality varies from 0 to 22% versus 2.1 to 18.6% outside Africa associated with New York Heart Association Functional Class IV as the most common significant risk factor for early deaths in all series in the World, including Africa.

Keywords: chronic constrictive pericarditis, epidemiology, etiology, diagnosis, pericardiectomy

1. Definition

Constrictive pericarditis is a reduction or a quasi-absence of heart distension because of a chronic inflammatory, thickened, and compressive pericardium.

2. Historical remark

Pericardium and pericardial diseases, especially constrictive pericarditis, have always been a concern for physicians and surgeons in cardiovascular field. Some remarkable landmarks [1, 2] are as follows: the first anatomical description of the pericardium has been done by Hippocrates in 460 BC. Centuries after, surgical treatment started in the seventeenth century by Riolan, who performed

IntechOpen

a pericardotomy for an effusion in 1649. Then, Vieussens, some years later in 1679 and 1715, observed some cases of pericardial adhesions; from that step, the concept of constrictive pericarditis was born. Afterward, in 1728, Lancisi confirmed the existence of constrictive pericarditis and its risks such as cardiac compression and death via necropsy studies. Those observations were also mentioned by Morgagni (1761), Senac (1749), Laennec (1819), and Cheevers (1842). Clinical patterns related to the right atrium and ventricle compression, mainly as the most important source in the compression process, has been emphasized by Wilkes (1870). Based on anatomical findings, clinical pictures were then clarified: Kussmaul (1873) pointed out the venous pressure elevation in case of constrictive pericarditis; Pick (1896) described a new entity named "Pericarditis pseudocirrhosis of the liver." Since then, Pick Syndrome was recognized as a component of constrictive pericarditis clinical presentation. From that, surgical treatment was considered as the most efficient therapy for releasing heart compression due to pericardium thickness and fibrosis. By then, Rhen and Sauerbruck (1913) in Germany, Hallopeau in France (1921), Schmieden and Fisher (1926) in Germany, Churchill (1929) and Beck (1931) in USA performed the first cases of pericardiectomy for constrictive pericarditis successfully.

3. Anatomy and function of the pericardium

The pericardium is a solid fibro-serous sac that maintains the heart in the anterior mediastinum in a closed thoracic cavity called the "pericardial cavity." The pericardium has two main components: (1) an external, fibrous pericardium ensuring the fixity of the pericardium and (2) an internal serous pericardium with two principal layers: the visceral and the parietal pericardium. In a normal heart, the parietal and visceral pericardium release the pericardial cavity filled with a fluid up to 50 ml allowing easy systolic and diastolic heart movements. Pericardium prevents the heart from inflammation, infection, damage, and excessive dilatation; it also ensures heart stabilization and anchoring [1–3].

4. Pathophysiology

In case of constrictive pericarditis, restricted diastolic heart distensibility does exist and may provoke a right and a left ventricular preload decrease with a reduction of stroke volume and cardiac output [2, 3]. In Africa, we use to face on late clinical presentation of patients with massive pericardial thickness and calcifications inducting myocardial atrophy, fibrosis, and severe systolic dysfunction that significantly affect the results after pericardiectomy.

Key observations are described:

1. Impairment of ventricular distensibility and filling coexisting with ventricular stroke volume reduction.

2. Abnormal rapid diastolic ventricular filling and abnormal venous pressure elevation followed by an early diastolic ventricular dip.

3. High diastolic plateau due to a small expansion of the ventricular volume at the late diastolic period.

All those consequences determine the so called "Dip-and-plateau waveform."

5. Epidemiology and etiology

Classically, constrictive pericarditis appears as a complication of acute or effusive pericarditis. From Yadav's study [4], approximately 9% of patients with acute pericarditis will contract a pericardial constriction. In Africa, the frequency of acute pericarditis varies widely with geographical location ranging from 2 to 11.3% among patients admitted in a hospital for cardiovascular diseases [5–7]; it affects mostly young male population with an average age between 26 and 42 years old and tuberculosis as the most frequent etiology from 33 to 69.5% in sub-Saharan Africa [5, 6, 8]. Over the past decades, the incidence of tuberculous pericarditis has risen up because of the HIV epidemic in sub-Saharan Africa [8, 9]. Noubiap et al. [10] have reported a comprehensive understanding of the epidemiology of pericardial diseases in Africa confirming clearly that tuberculosis remains as the leading cause of pericardial diseases in African Resource-Limited Settings with poor outcome marked by a mortality rate between 18 and 25% including a very high one of 40% within 6 months among patients with HIV/AIDS positive. However, pericardial tuberculosis frequency is variable according to authors such as Mayosi [11] and Thwaites [12] who found, respectively, pericardial tuberculosis in 69.5% of cases admitted for pericardiocentesis and in 10% of all hospitalized patients with heart failure. Moreover, the risk for developing constrictive is very high for tuberculosis or purulent pericarditis: 20–30% and in almost all the cases of tuberculous pericarditis as reported by Gupta [13]. In their prospective study on 500 consecutive cases, Imazzio et al. [14] have demonstrated that the evolution from non-constrictive pericarditis to constriction is different according to pericarditis etiology: the risk of constriction is greater for bacterial etiologies (tuberculosis or purulent pericarditis) than viral or idiopathic acute pericarditis; the incidence rate of constriction is, respectively, 31.65 cases per 1000 person-years for tuberculous pericarditis and 52.74 person-years for purulent pericarditis versus 0.76 person-years for viral or idiopathic pericarditis. The same observation has been described by Permanyer-Miralda et al. [15] in a prospective study of patients with occurrence of constriction in 56 and 35% of patients with tuberculous and purulent pericarditis, respectively, and in 17% of patients with neoplastic pericarditis after an acute pericarditis. In Africa, and in literature overall, the epidemiological pattern, incidence, and prevalence of CCP are not well elucidated. Nevertheless, it is known that tuberculosis is the most frequent etiology of constrictive pericarditis in Africa and emerging countries (40–90%) [16] versus other rare etiology in our practice such as constrictive pericarditis after surgery. In a recent study, Gaudino et al. [17] have concluded their study insisting on the fact that constrictive pericarditis after surgery has its own pathophysiological characteristics, but we still be ignorant on its real origin and pathogenesis. Therefore, we should be vigilant and keep in mind that any cardiac symptoms without explanation must be suspected and be treated surgically as soon as possible if there is any doubt of pericardial constriction.

6. Diagnosis

In African countries [18–26], the diagnosis of constrictive pericarditis is usually obvious for patients present late after the development of the constrictive process characterized mostly by advanced clinical manifestations of right-sided heart failure (50–100%), progressive New York Heart Association (NYHA) Functional Class III or IV (42–100%) associated with an evident antecedent pulmonary and extra-pulmonary tuberculosis such as tuberculous pericarditis (26–99%). Duration of illness prior to surgery may range from 1 month to 25 years with an average of 15 or 30 months found, respectively, by Ali et al. [26] and Yangni-Angate et al. [21].

Generally, male gender predominance is noted (60–80%), patients have an average age below 40 years; for instance in Morocco (32 years) [18], Ghana (33 years) [22], Senegal (23 years) [20], Gabon (36 years) [23], Cote d'Ivoire (28.8 years) [21], and Ethiopia (24.3 years) [26]. Main clinical findings often due to severe constriction include: hepatomegaly (74–100%), raised jugular venous pressure (76–100%), hepato-jugular reflux (67–100%), ascite (50–76%), peripheral edema (46–79%), complete "Pick Syndrome"(50–76%). Kussmaul sign is less detected (9.8%). In African setting, frequent radiographical findings at chest X-ray are as follows: enlarged cardiothoracic ratio or cardiomegaly (88–47%), calcifications (36–52.5%), and pleural effusion (44–63%); electrocardiography shows invariable modifications such as low QRS voltage (32.5–82.5%), atrial fibrillation (18–46%), and T wave abnormality up to 87.5%. Echocardiography is largely available and is useful for accurate assessment in revealing in most cases a thickened pericardium (56 and 100%), pericardial calcifications in 30.2%, 47.4% of cases according to authors and left ventricular septal motion abnormality (63.6%) with reduced ejection fraction below 0.60 in Rabat, Morocco [19]; cardiac catheterization performed only in a very few centers [21, 24, 25, 27] documents elevation and equalization of diastolic heart pressures with the typical dip-plateau waveform of constrictive pericarditis and evaluate the stroke volume, cardiac output, and myocardial systolic function. It still prevails to be the most final diagnostic assessment in sub-Saharan Africa. In his study, Yangni-Angate et al. [21] reported that cardiac catheterization confirmed a dip-and-plateau (square root sign), an equalization of end-diastolic pressures in right and/or left cardiac chambers ranged between 10 and 40 mmHg, a mean cardiac index (CI): 2.3 $l/min/m^2$ (extremes: 1.3–3.6). From this author, the constriction was limited to the right cardiac cavities called right constriction ($n = 54$, 45%) or to the right and left cardiac cavities called bilateral constriction ($n = 66$, 55%) and hemodynamic parameters and cineangiograms confirmed the diagnosis of pericardial constriction in all the patients. Omboga in Nairobi [25] showed the same observation with elevation of intracardial pressures in all cases, raised mean right atrium, end-diastolic right and left ventricular, and elevated mean pulmonary artery pressures at 18, 18, 20, and 27mmHg, respectively. Other imaging studies such as computed tomography and magnetic resonance imaging are rarely prescribed because they are inexistent usually. Those modern imaging techniques could be heavily useful in diagnosing constrictive pericarditis. When done, pericardial biopsy can be contributive for constrictive pericarditis etiology. Laboratory investigations regarding protein-losing enteropathy in patients with chronic constrictive pericarditis are not yet done for Africans. Differential diagnosis is always considered, and distinction from both constrictive pericarditis and restrictive cardiomyopathy due to endomyocardial fibrosis is really the usual situation to be clarified. Endomyocardial fibrosis (EMF) is a tropical heart disease with fibrous endocardial lesions lying in the right and/or the left ventricle. Endoventricular fibrosis is shown and confirmed in all cases by bi-dimensional echocardiography and angiocardiography [28].

7. Natural history

Constrictive pericarditis occurs mostly in our African context after a non-diagnosed, untreated tuberculous or pyogenic pericarditis or even as a sequel of a treated tuberculous pericarditis. Constrictive process starts with an acute pericarditis; then a subacute and chronic pericarditis marked in most of the cases by a fusion of the two layers of the pericardium and an occlusion of the pericardial cavity [3].

The delay from onset clinical symptoms to constriction is widely flexible from 1 month to 10 years even 25 years [2].

8. Surgical treatment

When diagnosis of constrictive pericarditis is confirmed and surgery is indicated, a pericardiectomy should not be delayed; surgery remains the only efficient and comprehensive treatment option. Pericardiectomy is frequently performed via a median sternotomy approach or a left anterolateral thoracotomy approach; it may be partial or complete. From the African teams' surgical experiences, cardiopulmonary bypass has not been used in all cases and excellent early surgical outcomes were reported.

9. Early outcomes and risk factors for early deaths

9.1 From cardiac centers in Africa

Yangni-Angate in Cote d'Ivoire [21], in his retrospective study related to 120 patients with CCP who underwent pericardiectomy through a median sternotomy approach (n = 117; 97.5%) found 15 early deaths (12.5%); the cause of hospital deaths was due to a low cardiac output (n = 12) and to a hepatic failure (n = 3). Class III or IV (NYHA) ($p = 0.01$), mitral regurgitation ($p < 0.05$), persistent a diastolic syndrome after surgery ($p < 0.05$) and low cardiac index ($p < 0.02$) were the important risk factors (**Table 1**). Age, size of cardiac X-ray silhouette, right and left ventricular diastolic pressures, ejection fraction, atrial fibrillation, and pericardial calcifications had no impact on early survival (**Table 2**).

Tettey in Ghana [22] reviewed the surgical management of constructive pericarditis and the post-operative challenges of 11 patients who had pericardiectomy via a median sternotomy in all patients with no early mortality and a significant improvement of functional capacity of all of the patients followed-up.

Mutyaba in South Africa [24] through a retrospective study of 121 patients who had undergone total (n = 105; 88.2%) or partial (n = 14; 11.8%) pericardiectomy for constrictive pericarditis at Groote Schuur Hospital, noted an early mortality of 14% (n = 14) mainly due to a low cardiac output syndrome. In this work, it has been statistically attested that serum sodium and pre-operative New York Heart Association Class IV versus combined Class I–III were independent predictors of early mortality. He also showed that early mortality after pericardiectomy was not influenced by HIV status and that of New York Heart Association Functional Class IV and hyponatremia were predictable factor for early mortality after pericardiectomy.

Ali in Ethiopia [26] has done a retrospective study at the Thoracic Surgical Unit, Tikur Anbessa Hospital, Department of Surgery, Medical Faculty, Addis Ababa University, Addis Ababa on 19 patients who underwent pericardiectomy for CCP by a median sternotomy approach (n = 15; 79%) often. One early post-operative mortality was registered. The author emphasized the benefit of pericardiectomy in terms of physical exercise improvement.

Ondo N'Dong in Gabon [23] has published his series on 18 patients with constrictive pericarditis treated surgically. All of them underwent a partial pericardiectomy via a left anterior thoracic incision in 17 patients and a median sternotomy incision in 1 patient. Four patients died in the early post-operative period due to low cardiac output; this study revealed pre-operative severe heart failure as a principal predictable risk factor for early death after pericardiectomy. This finding has been also noted In Rabat, Morocco by Nzondo [19]; in Fes, Morocco by Hind [18] and in Senegal by Ciss [20].

Nzondo [19] has retrospectively analyzed 11 patients who had undergone partial pericardiectomy via a median sternotomy approach for constrictive pericarditis. Early mortality was of 9.1% related to acute heart and multi-organs failure. Hind in

Author	Country	Study period	Cases (n)	Aetiology	Early deaths (%)	Causes of deaths	Early risk factors
Omboga et al. [25]	KENYA	1973–1981	51	TB (30%) Idiopathic (70%)	8.5	• Pulmonary embolism (n=3) • Massive haemorrhage (n=1)	–
Yangni–Angate et al. [21]	Cote d'Ivoire	1977–2012	120	TB (99%)	12.5	• Low cardiac output (n=12) • Hepatic failure (n=3)	• Class III or IV (NYHA) • Low cardiac index • Mitral regurgitation • Persistent diastolic post-operative syndrome
Ondo N'Dong et al. [23]	Gabon	1986–1999	18	TB (50%) Idiopathic (33%) Infection (17%)	22.2	Low cardiac output (n=4)	Class IV (NYHA)
Mutyaba et al. [24]	South Africa	1990–2012	121	TB (91%) Idiopathic (5%) Miscellaneous (4%)	14	Low cardiac output (n=11) Acute kidney injury (n=6)	Class IV (NYHA)
Zamani et al. [27]	Morocco	1994–2009	23	TB (43%) Idiopathic (57%)	17	Low cardiac output (n=2) Severe dysarythmia (n=1) Haemorrhage (n=1)	Class IV (NYHA)
Ali et al. [26]	Ethiopia	1996–2005	19	TB (31.6%) Infection (10.5%) Miscellaneous (67.9%)	5.3	–	–
Ciss et al. [20]	Senegal	1996–2008	32	TB (63.6%)	6.25	Low cardiac output (n=1)	Class IV (NYHA)
Nzondo et al. [19]	Morocco	1996–2010	11	TB (45.5%) Idiopathic (54.5%)	9.1	Low cardiac output (n=1)	Class IV (NYHA)
Tettey et al. [22]	Ghana	2000–2004	11	TB (63.6%)	0		
Hind et al. [18]	Morocco	2003–2013	43	TB (58%) Idiopathic (48%)	4.6	Low cardiac output (n=2)	Class IV (NYHA)

TB: Tuberculosis.

Table 1.
Surgical early results after pericardiectomy for chronic constrictive pericarditis.

Risk factors for immediate deaths	Alive (n = 105)		Deceased (n = 15)		P
	Average	Extremes	Average	Extremes	
Age (years)	30.4 ± 16.6	10–51	28.4 ± 10.1	8–46	0.09
CTR	0.55 ± 0.05	0.45–0.70	0.53 ± 0.3	0.50–0.59	0.34
RVEDP	20.6 ± 7.8	7–40	16.2 ± 10.3	15–40	0.12
LVEDP	20.1 ± 6.1	10–30	24.6 ± 7.7	16–35	0.07
EF	50.4 ± 16	31–67	54.3 ± 5	49–59	0.24
CI	2.42 ± 0.7	1.3–3.6	1.63 ± 0.2	1.4–2	0.02
WPAP	20.6 ± 9.9	10–40	25 ± 10.4	18–37	0.36
SPAP	27.3 ± 11.1	21–66	38.2 ± 17.9	21–66	0.08
Functional class NYHA III–IV	42/105		15/15		0.01
Atrial fibrillation	18/105		3/15		0.10
Calcifications	54/105		6/15		0.07
Mitral insufficiency	6/105		9/15		0.00
Persistence of post-operative constriction	9/105		5/15		0.00
Bilateral constriction	61/105		15/15		0.04

CTR, cardiothoracic ratio; RVEDP, right ventricle end-diastolic pressure; SPAP, systolic pulmonary arterial pressure; WPAP, wedged pulmonary artery pressure; LVEPD, left ventricle end-diastolic pressure; CI, cardiac index; EF, ejection fraction.

Table 2.
Risk Factors for immediate deaths after pericardiectomy for constrictive chronic pericarditis—from Yangni-Angate et al. study [21].

Fes, Morocco [18] on a study of 43 patients with constrictive pericarditis focused on 41 who had a partial pericardiectomy through a median sternotomy approach; hospital mortality was 4.6% (n = 2).

Finally, Ciss et al. [20] in their study on 32 patients with constrictive pericarditis undergoing partial pericardiectomy via a median sternotomy approach reported an early mortality of 6.25% in 2 patients out of 32 caused by hemodynamic and severe instability added to a poor NYHA functional class pre-operatively.

Omboga in Nairobi [25] in his study of 47 patients out of 51 who underwent surgery through median sternotomy (82.9%) and left lateral thoracic (17.1%) approaches has mentioned 8.5% of hospital mortality not due to acute failure as mentioned in previous studies in Africa but attributable to massive hemorrhage in the operative table (n = 1) and pulmonary embolism (n = 3) secondary to deep venous thrombosis.

None of African teams mentioned above used robotic approach; this minimally invasive modern approach seems to be less painful, more adequate for a complete release of the pericardial constriction [29].

9.2 From worldwide outside Africa

Compared to African series, where the most common etiology of CCP is TB, in developed world CCP etiology profile is different with idiopathic as most frequent. However, there is no significant difference among either surgical operative approach and hospital mortality or risk factors for early deaths. This fact is on the same line with McCaughan's consideration cited by Kirklin and Barratt-Boyes [2] who demonstrated in 1985 that most of early deaths are due to acute heart failure and that of pre-operative NYHA class III and IV are significant risk factor for early death after pericardiectomy as noted in African surgical experiences. Chowdhury et al. [30] in a study including 338 patients (85.6%) who underwent total pericardiectomy (group I), and 57 patients (14.4%) undergoing partial pericardiectomy (group II), has demonstrated better perioperative and late mortality rates after total pericardiectomy; in addition, duration of symptoms, advanced functional class, partial pericardiectomy, pre-operative high right atrial pressure, hyperbilirubinemia, renal dysfunction, atrial fibrillation, pericardial calcification, thoracotomy approach, were significant risk factors for death.

In a recent study from Porta-Sanchez in Spain [31], 140 consecutive patients who underwent pericardiectomy for constrictive pericarditis over a 34-year period in a single center were analyzed. Most frequent etiology found was idiopathic in 76 patients (54%). Median sternotomy was done in all patients. Perioperative mortality was 11%. There was no difference in mortality between etiologies.

Mayo Clinic Experience with pericardiectomy for constrictive pericarditis over eight decades [32] related to 1071 pericardiectomies in 1066 individual patients. Patients were divided into two intervals: an historical (pre-1990) group ($n = 259$) and a contemporary (1990–2013) group ($n = 807$). This study showed a significant change in constrictive pericarditis etiology with a similar overall survival over decades and a significant decrease of 30-day mortality from 13.5% in the historical era to 5.2% in the contemporary era ($p < 0.001$). Another article from North America with no significant disparity is the Montreal Heart Institute Experience over a 20-year period [33]; it involved 99 consecutive patients with constrictive pericarditis; idiopathic was the most frequent etiology (61%) and hospital mortality 7.9% after isolated pericardiectomy.

Busha et al. [34] revealed an higher mortality death of 18.6% after pericardiectomy in 97 consecutive patients with constrictive pericarditis and no different risk factors for early death such as reduced left ventricular ejection fraction (LVEF) (35% < LVEF <55%) and right ventricular dilatation on multivariable analysis. He also found no difference in early mortality between patients with isolated pericardiectomy and those with concomitant surgery ($p = 0.62$).

10. Late outcomes

In African context, lack of substantial late outcomes after pericardiectomy is observed due to a significant number of patients lost to follow-up in general; however, in his series from Cote d'ivoire, Yangni-Angate [21], after an average follow-up of 4 years (extremes: 1–10 years), no late death was observed. A functional class I or II (NYHA) was mentioned in all survivors. Among them, those who underwent cardiac catheterization late post-operatively, a significant reduction even a normalization of the right and/or the left ventricular end-diastolic pressures, of the pulmonary capillary wedge pressure ($p < 0.05$) and of the right atrial pressure ($p < 0.05$) and absence of the dip-and-plateau after pericardiectomy were certified (**Table 3**).

Significant reduction of right atrial mean pressure from 17 ± 6 mmHg preoperatively to 7.1 ± 4.2 mmHg after pericardiectomy for CCP has been also shown by an African team work published by Zamani in Rabat, Morrocco [27].

A similar experience as African teams series has been published by Bicer et al. [35] with a predominance of tuberculous constrictive pericarditis (48.8%); other etiologies were: idiopathic (31.9%), malignancy (6.4%), prior cardiac surgery (4.3%), non-tuberculosis bacterial infections (4.3%), radiotherapy (2.1%), uremia (2.1%), and post-traumatic (2.1%). They had performed pericardiectomy in all patients via a sternotomy approach with a very low early mortality of 2.1%, while

Hemodynamic measurements	Average		Extremes		P
	Preop.	Postop.	Preop.	Postop.	
RAP	16	7.4	10–36	5–10	0.04
RVEDP	21	10	7–40	5–15	0.02
SPAP	29	23	8–66	17–30	0.09
WPAP	21	14	10–40	9–19	0.00
LVEDP	21	13	10–35	4.5–20	0.02
CI	2.3	2.7	1.2–36	1.92–3.5	0.15

Significant ($P < 0.05$); Non-significant ($P \geq 0.05$); Preop., Pre-operative; Postop., Post-operative; RAP, right atrial pressure; RVEDP, right ventricle end-diastolic pressure; SPAP, systolic pulmonary arterial pressure; WPAP, wedged pulmonary artery pressure; LVEPD, left ventricle end-diastolic pressure; CI, cardiac index.

Table 3.
Comparison of hemodynamic measurements: pre-operative versus post-operative in patients who underwent pericardiectomy for chronic constrictive pericarditis—from Yangni-Angate et al. study [21].

late mortality was 23.4%, and actuarial survival rates at 1, 5, 10 years were 91, 85, and 81%, respectively. Those rates are closed to the Montreal Heart Institute experience [33] characterized by tolerable long-term clinical outcome: 79% of patients were in NYHA class I or II post-operatively with an overall survival rate of 87% at 5 years and 78% at 10 years. At 10 years survival, Bicer et al. [35] estimated rate was worse (64%) because of poor prognosis of pericardiectomy after constrictive pericarditis post-mediastinal irradiation.

In a 24-year experience on pericardiectomy in patients with constrictive pericarditis, based on Kaplan-Meier survival curves demonstration, Szaboa et al. [36] have confirmed poor prognosis of post-irradiation constrictive pericardiectomy and shown better and comparable long-term survival after in other etiologies as idiopathic tuberculosis myocardial infarction, and uremia; the author noted no survival after 5 years with post-radiation constrictive pericarditis; it is widely accepted radiation etiology is a negative factor affecting long-term survival results as well indicated by Nishimura in Japanese population [37] and Avgerinos et al. [38]. On his study related to 46 patients with a mean age of 59 years and various classic etiologies, Nishumuna et al. [37] have described the very high severity of radiation etiology with death within only 1 year after pericardiectomy confirming overall literature results.

Avgerinos et al. [38] reported his 36 patients study who underwent pericardiectomy for constrictive pericarditis over 15 years; he has no hospital mortality and 1-, 5-, 10-, and 15-year survival rates were 97.2, 94.6, 86.5, and 78.3%, respectively; he fund risk factors for increased long-term mortality such as: pre-operative heart failure, elevated pre-operative total bilirubin (>2.7 mg/dl, hazard ratio 6.8, $p = 0.02$), and elevated creatinine (>1.4 mg/dl, hazard ratio 3.1, $p = 0.05$). Subsequently, he demonstrated from Kaplan-Meier survival analysis a significant decrease in survival of all the patients with post-radiation etiology associated ($p = 0.05$) or with impaired cardiac, hepatic or renal dysfunction.

According to Porta-Sanchez et al. [31], from a Cox-regression analysis in his study, age at surgery, advanced New York Heart Association Functional Class (III–IV) and previous acute idiopathic pericarditis were associated with increased mortality during follow-up ranging from 0.1 to 33.0 years with a mean follow-up of 12 years.

Predictor factors of prognosis and mortality after pericardiectomy have been largely documented by many studies; one of them from Kang [39] has even stipulated that an echocardiographical measurement of higher early diastolic mitral inflow velocity in predicting mortality after pericardiectomy was 71 cm/s (sensitivity of 84.6% and specificity of 52.2%); that value may also be useful in predicting late survival ($p = 0.029$).

Because of satisfactory long-term results, pericardiectomy can be considered as a safe and efficient technical procedure [40]; it can be achieved in most cases with minimal hospital mortality, post-operative functional class significant improvement and substantial reduction of heart diastolic pressures and absence of any recurrence if completely performed.

Author details

Koffi Herve Yangni-Angate
Chairman, Department of Cardiovascular and Thoracic Surgery, Bouake Teaching Hospital and University, Bouake, Cote d'Ivoire

*Address all correspondence to: yangniangate@yahoo.fr

IntechOpen

© 2019 The Author(s). Licensee IntechOpen. This chapter is distributed under the terms of the Creative Commons Attribution License (http://creativecommons.org/licenses/by/3.0), which permits unrestricted use, distribution, and reproduction in any medium, provided the original work is properly cited. (cc) BY

References

[1] Paul EA, Hassan N. The pericardium. In: Sabiston DC, editor. Surgery of the Chest. 5th ed. Philadelphia: Saunders; 1990. pp. 1230-1249

[2] Kirklin J, Barrat-Boyes B. Pericardial disease. In: Cardiac Surgery. 3rd ed. Philadelphia: Elsevier (USA); 2003. pp. 1779-1795

[3] Lorell BH, Braunwald E. Pericardial disease. In: Heart Disease. A Textbook of Cardiovascular Medicine. 3rd ed. Philadelphia: Saunders; 1988. pp. 1484-1534

[4] Yadav NK, Siddique MS. Constrictive Pericarditis. StatPearls Publishing; 2018

[5] Pio M, Afassinou YM, Pessinaba S, Mossi KE, et al. Effusive pericarditis: Clinical and etiological aspects. Lomé Medecine et Santé Tropicales. 2016;**26**:92-96

[6] Magassouba S. Péricadites: Prise en charde et pronostic au service de chirurgie thoracique de l'hôpital national donka. Étude de 19 cas Université Gamal El Nasser de Conakry - Doctorat 2012. Available from: https://www.memoireonline.com › Biologie et Médecine

[7] Maiga MBH. Epidemiology of acute pericarditis on 76 cases. Cardiology Unit, Bamako University Teaching Hospital, Point G. 2005 indexmedicus.afro.who.int/iah/fulltext/Thesis

[8] Yameogo AA, Kyelem CG, Nikiéma Z, Birba E, et al. Les péricardites tuberculeuses au Centre Hospitalier Universitaire de Bobo-Dioulasso, Burkina Faso. The Pan African Medical Journal. 2012;**16**:1-5

[9] Reuter H et al. Epidemiology of Pericardial Effusions at a Large Academic Hospital in South Africa. Vol. 133. Cambridge University Press; 2005. pp. 393-399

[10] Noubiap JJ, Noubiap JJN, Agbor VN, Ndoadoumgue AL, et al. Epidemiology of pericardial diseases in Africa: A systematic scoping review in Heart (British Cardiac Society). 2018. DOI: 10.1136/heartjnl-2018-313922

[11] Mayosi B. Chapter 31—Tuberculous pericarditis and myocarditis in adults and children. In: Tuberculosis. A Comprehensive Clinical Reference. 2009. pp. 351-360. DOI: 10.1016/B978-1-4160-3988-4.00031-7

[12] Thwaites G. Tuberculosis Manson's Tropical Infectious Diseases. 23rd ed2014. pp. 468-505. DOI: 10.1016/B978-0-7020-5101-2.00041-8

[13] Gupta P. Chapter 16 - The pericardium and its diseases cellular and molecular pathobiology. In: Cardiovascular Disease. 2014. pp. 297-314. DOI: 10.1016/B978-0-12-405206-2.00016-8

[14] Imazio M, Brucato A, Maestroni S, Cumetti D, Belli R, Trinchero R, et al. Risk of constrictive pericarditis after acute pericarditis. Circulation. 2011;**124**:1270-1275

[15] Permanyer-Miralda G, Sagristà-Sauleda J, Soler-Soler J. Primary acute pericardial disease: A prospective series of 231 consecutive patients. The American Journal of Cardiology. 1985;**56**:623-630

[16] Mutyaba AK, Mayosi BM. Emerging Countries and Tuberculosis Constriction Expert Analysis. American College of Cardiology. 2016. Available from: https://www.acc.org/emerging-countries-and-tuberculosis-constriction

[17] Gaudino M, Anselmi A, Pavone N, Massetti M. Constrictive pericarditis after cardiac surgery. The Annals of Thoracic Surgery. 2013;**95**:731-736

[18] Hind D. Chronic constrictive pericardits: Experience of cardiovascular unit(A): 43 cases. Faculty of Medicine and Pharmacy, Sidi Mohamed Ben Abdellah University, Fès. Thesis N° 110/14; 2014. scolarite.fmpusmba.ac.ma/cdim/mediatheque/e_theses/110-14.pdf

[19] Nzondo MLK. Chronic constrictive pericardits: Experience of cardiovascular unit (B):11 cases. Faculty of Medicine and Pharmacy, Mohamed V University. Rabat Thesis N° 108; 2011

[20] Ciss AG, Dieng PA, Ba S, et al. Outcomes of surgery in constrictive pericarditis in Dakar. African Journal of Surgery. 2012;**3**:139-142

[21] Yangni-Angate KH, Tanauh Y, Meneas C, Diby F, et al. Surgical experience on chronic constrictive pericarditis in African setting: Review of 35 years' experience in Cote d'Ivoire. Cardiovascular Diagnosis and Therapy. 2016;**6**(Suppl. 1):S13-S19

[22] Tettey M, Sereboe L, Aniteye E, et al. Surgical management of constrictive pericarditis. Ghana Medical Journal. 2007;**41**:190-193

[23] Ondo N'Dong F, Mbamendane S, Ndong Assapi M, et al. Surgical treatment of chronic constrictive pericarditis at Libreville. African Annals of Thoracic and Cardiovascular Surgeons. 2005;**1**:15-18

[24] Mutyaba AK, Balkaran S, Cloete R, Du Plessis N, Badri M, Brink J, et al. Constrictive pericarditis requiring pericardiectomy at Groote Schuur Hospital, Cape Town, South Africa: Causes and perioperative outcomes in the HIV era (1990-2012). The Journal of Thoracic and Cardiovascular Surgery. 2014;**148**(6):3058-3065

[25] Omboga PN. Chronic Constrictive Pericarditis. UoN Repository, University of Nairobi. Available from: Erepository.uonbi.ac.ke/.../Omboga_Chronic%20Constrictive%20P

[26] Ali A, Biluts H, Bekele A. Experience of pericardiectomy in Tikur Anbessa University Hospital. Ethiopia East and Central African Journal of Surgery. 2007;**1**:114-119

[27] Zamani O. Surgery of chronic constrictive pericardits: About 23 cases. Faculty of Medicine and Pharmacy, Mohamed V University. Rabat Thesis N° 239; 2009

[28] Yangni-Angate KH, Ayegnon G, Fl D, et al. Bilateral endomyocardial fibrosis in children: An Ivorian surgical experience. African Journal of Paediatric Surgery. 2007;**4**(2):64-67

[29] Maciolek K, Asfaw ZE, Krienbring DJ, Arnsdorf SE, Balkhy HH. Robotic endoscopic off-pump total pericardiectomy in constrictive pericarditis. Innovations. 2016;**11**:134-137

[30] Chowdhury UK, Subramaniam GK, Kumar AS, Airan B, et al. Pericardiectomy for constrictive pericarditis: A clinical, echocardiographic, and hemodynamic evaluation of two surgical techniques. The Annals of Thoracic Surgery. 2006;**81**:522-530

[31] Porta-Sanchez A, Sagrista-Sauleda J, Ferreira-Gonzalez I, Torrents-Fernandez A, et al. Constrictive pericarditis: Etiologic spectrum, patterns of clinical presentation, prognostic factors, and long-term follow-up. Revista Española de Cardiología. 2015;**68**:1092-1100

[32] Murashita T, Schaff HV, Daly RC, Oh JK, et al. Experience with pericardiectomy for constrictive pericarditis over eight decades. The Annals of Thoracic Surgery. 2017;**104**:742-750

[33] Vistarini N, Chen C, Mazine A, Bouchard D. Pericardiectomy for

constrictive pericarditis: 20 years of experience at the Montreal Heart Institute. The Annals of Thoracic Surgery. 2015;**100**(1):107-113

[34] Busch C, Penov K, Amorim PA, Garbade J, et al. Risk factors for mortality after pericardiectomy for chronic constrictive pericarditis in a large single-centre cohort. European Journal of Cardio-Thoracic Surgery. 2015;**48**:e110-e116

[35] Biçer M, Özdemir B, Kan I, Yüksel A, et al. Long-term outcomes of pericardiectomy for constrictive pericarditis. Journal of Cardiothoracic Surgery. 2015;**10**:177. DOI: 10.1186/s13019-015-0385-8

[36] Szabóa G, Schmacka B, Bulutc C, Soósb P, et al. Constrictive pericarditis: Risks, aetiologies and outcomes after total pericardiectomy: 24 years of experience. European Journal of Cardio-Thoracic Surgery. 2013;**44**:1023-1028

[37] Nishimura S, Izumi C, Amano M, Imamura S, et al. Long-term clinical outcomes and prognostic factors after pericardiectomy for constrictive pericarditis in a Japanese population. Circulation Journal. 2017;**81**:206-212

[38] Avgerinos D, Rabitnokov Y, Worku B, Neragi-Miandoab S, et al. Fifteen-year experience and outcomes of pericardiectomy for constrictive pericarditis. Journal of Cardiac Surgery. 2014;**29**:434-438

[39] Kang SH, Song JM, Kim M, Choo SJ, et al. Prognostic predictors in pericardiectomy for chronic constrictive pericarditis. The Journal of Thoracic and Cardiovascular Surgery. 2014;**147**(2):598-605. DOI: 10.1016/j.jtcvs.2013.01.022. Epub: 2013 Feb 4

[40] Nachum E, Sternik L, Kassif Y, Raanani E, et al. Surgical pericardiectomy for constrictive pericarditis: A single tertiary center experience. The Thoracic and Cardiovascular Surgeon. 2018. DOI: 10.1055/s-0038-1645869

Chapter 5

Pericardial Diseases: Surgery for Pericardial Effusion

Ing Xiang Soo

Abstract

Management of pericardial effusion is a common topic for cardiothoracic surgeons. From a surgeon's perspective, we would review and evaluate patients for surgical drainage. Besides discussing the frequent indications for performing pericardial window creation, we would go through the decision-making process during the perioperative management of these patients who might be critically ill. For example, regardless of whether surgery is for diagnostic or therapeutic reasons, the risks of surgery must be weighed against the benefits including the odds of quality of life across a reasonable life expectancy.

Keywords: pericardial window, surgical drainage

1. Introduction

Management of pericardial effusion is a common topic for cardiothoracic surgeons. In this chapter, we will discuss the common etiologies referred for surgical management. From a surgeon's perspective, we would review how to evaluate patients for surgical drainage, as well as the frequent indications for performing pericardial window creation. Technically, surgery is rather straightforward compared to other procedures done by cardiothoracic surgeons; however, it requires lots of decision-making experience during the perioperative management of these patients who might be critically ill. For example, regardless of whether surgery is for diagnostic or therapeutic reasons, the risks of surgery must be weighed against the benefits including the odds of quality of life across a reasonable life expectancy.

Other discussion points will include anterior thoracotomy technique vs. video-assisted thoracoscopic surgery (VATS) approach. Other technical points include identifying the phrenic nerve and removing adequate pericardial tissue anterior to the nerve to avoid risk of recurrent pericardial effusions.

2. Reasons requiring surgical drainage

2.1 Neoplastic

The common etiologies encountered in surgery for pericardial effusion can be broadly classified into neoplastic, infective, and reactive. For neoplastic causes, frequently malignant pericardial effusion can manifest after tumor involvement of the pericardium. Majority of this type of effusion will be from hematogenous spread, whereby primary tumors of the pericardium are rare [1]. Occasionally, pericardium effusions can result from local spread of thymic malignancy and even myocardial tumor-like lymphoma. We will discuss the rationale for proceeding with therapeutic surgical drainage for this group of patients later, as this involves a careful consideration of their long-term prognosis.

2.2 Infective

Another etiology of pericardial effusions will include infectious causes. Even though rare in this day and age due to the use of antibiotics, infection of the pericardial space is a consideration in immunocompromised patients. These groups of patients can be rather septic from this deep-lying infection, especially if the source is bacterial in origin. In areas where tuberculosis is still prevalent, infection involving the pericardial cavity has been reported [2]. Treatment with the appropriate antibiotics can then be optimized when drainage has been achieved and the correct causative organism identified. The role of the surgeon here is to assist in surgical drainage for both therapeutic and diagnostic reasons. Occasionally, smaller bore drains inserted percutaneously are unable to reduce septic foci, and surgery is required for source control. However, unlike creating a permanent window for drainage into the pleural space in cases of malignant effusions, I would be less inclined to do so for infective causes. This is to avoid contaminating the pleural space with infection.

2.3 Traumatic

For trauma-induced pericardial effusion, most surgeons would suggest surgical exploration rather than conservative approach. This is because in the acute setting, most patients are unstable with multiple injuries, and they would require urgent surgery to exclude ongoing bleeding into the pericardial cavity. The resultant tamponade is rapidly fatal unless drainage and hemostasis are quickly established. Any blunt or penetrating injury in the cardiac box (bounded by both nipple lines laterally, the clavicles superiorly and the costal margin inferiorly) must be viewed with a high index of suspicion that there is myocardial injury. Opinion is divided between the left anterior thoracotomy incision and the sternotomy incision. The sternotomy approach is safer as it allows rapid access to the ascending aorta and vena cava if cardiopulmonary bypass is urgently required for repair of a heart chamber perforation. Left anterior thoracotomy avoids a bigger incision and the risk of sternal wound infection; however, if cardiopulmonary bypass is required, it may still require conversion to a sternotomy for better control. Another reason why traumatic pericardial effusion cannot be usually treated conservatively is the fact that most commonly the right ventricle is involved and this usually requires surgical repair.

2.4 Iatrogenic

Iatrogenic pericardial effusion can be caused by injury to any cardiac chamber or intra-pericardial injury to the superior vena cava. Especially if the patient is anticoagulated and symptomatic, urgent intervention is required. This may be in the form of an urgent pericardiocentesis to prevent impending cardiac tamponade [3]. If there is persistent drainage after pericardiocentesis or if it is unable to adequately decompress the pericardial cavity, emergency surgical drainage is indicated. The approach would be similar to that mentioned above, although I would recommend a sternotomy approach for better exposure and safety.

2.5 Others

Another common cause of pericardial effusion encountered by both thoracic and cardiac surgeons includes the broad group underreactive causes. This also covers the postcardiotomy pericarditis and Dressler's syndrome [4, 5]. It often occurs after cardiac surgery when the pericardium gets inflamed and produces pericardial fluid which cannot be reabsorbed fast enough. Drainage can be in the form of pericardiocentesis or open subxiphoid approach which avoids re-sternotomy. But for persistent pericardial effusions, creating a surgical window between the pericardial cavity and the pleural cavity is better suited for longer-term drainage.

I would classify unknown and idiopathic causes as underreactive. This is because despite clinical suspicion, some cases of pericardial effusion may not have a definitive diagnosis. Specimens of pericardium tissue and pericardial fluid obtained during surgery may only be labeled as inflammatory or even normal in appearance under the microscope. Hence, apart from knowing there is an inflammatory reason, the patient should be treated with other clinical inputs to achieve diagnosis. These causes which are also not exhaustive include uremic, auto-immune, drug-related and postradiation. However, despite not knowing the diagnosis, most of the time, surgical drainage is therapeutic and achieves the desired outcome of symptom relief.

3. Presurgical considerations

3.1 Indications

This is the portion that the art of medicine is needed more than the science. Being a surgeon, it would appear rather strange that I would advocate surgical drainage only if all other alternatives have been considered first. But my approach to surgical drainage of pericardial effusion is always to weigh the risks against the benefits. This is always the case in medicine and even more so in these patients who might be in extremis prior to surgery.

An ideal patient for surgical drainage would be one with good life expectancy despite advanced disease or cancer. I do not recommend surgical drainage for patients with less than 6 months of life expectancy. Surgical drainage is to improve long-term outcome and relief of symptoms in patients, so I would consider other forms of drainage for short-term belief.

3.2 Preoperative assessment

A great deal of effort is usually required to counsel the patient prior to any surgery for pericardial effusion. In fact, I take the most time to talk to this group of patients, even more than patients with other pathologies. This is because patients in this group tend to have multiple medical conditions and pro-morbidities which complicate surgery. Speaking to them and understanding their wishes and concerns is paramount. For example, if they are not affected functionally by the pericardial effusion, they may not want surgery especially if surgery is high risk and can lead to adverse outcomes which they might not accept.

The patient should not have any other contra-indications to general anesthesia. A good bedside assessment, which has been handed down from seniors, would be to check if the patient is able to lie completely flat with the head not elevated. This tells two things about the patient: firstly, the pericardial collection is not causing too much hemodynamic compromise that it is affecting venous return to the heart, and, secondly, it is to ensure there is no other pathology that could lead to his or her symptoms. It is an unwise clinical decision to operate and drain a pericardial effusion promising full relief of symptoms, where, for example, the symptoms are actually manifested from compression of the airway due to mediastinal disease.

3.3 Timing of surgery and long-term outcomes

The timing of creating a surgical pericardial window also varies widely. For the first presentations of pericardial effusions, surgery may not be always necessary after initial pericardiocentesis and resolution of pericardial effusions. As patients could be treated with chemotherapy or immunotherapy for their primary disease or the causative factors modified to reduce the risk of recurrent effusions, I do not recommend surgical drainage for all first presentations. However, once the effusion recurs, this increases the subsequent times that it continues to be recurrent; hence, I do advocate creating a pericardial window for this group of patients. As all other disease, discussion with the patients' primary physician or oncologist is advised to better optimize care.

Another issue which must be discussed with the patient is the likelihood of recurrent pericardial effusion despite surgical drainage. The risk of this recurring can be up to 16% in reported cases [6]. Of course there are technical pitfalls in this. For example, my preference is for an anterior thoracotomy rather than a subxiphoid approach. The latter could be under local anesthesia which sometimes is the only option in patients who are not candidates for general anesthesia. However, it has been reported to have higher failure rates [6]. This could be due to repositioning of the diaphragm closing off the window, leading to recurrent effusions. Other authors have found no significant differences between both techniques [7]. Most authors have described a 2–3 cm size of pericardium tissue to be excised [6–11]. Despite all efforts, recurrent pericardial effusions do occur, and patients should be counseled for this. It is not uncommon to see a loculated right pericardial effusion occurring after a left pericardial-pleural window (**Figures 1** and **2**). This can be contributed by intra-pericardial adhesions or disease which progress despite medical treatment. A redo pericardial window can be done in such patients and probably in my opinion, safer and more effective via a different side than the initial approach.

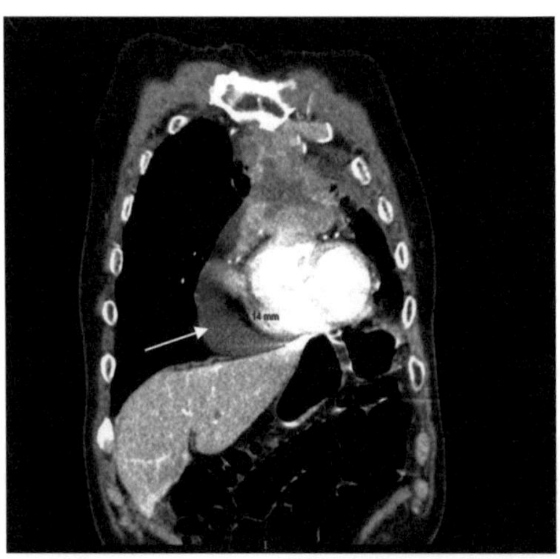

Figure 1.
Loculated right pericardial effusion (arrow). Patient had prior left pericardial-pleural window.

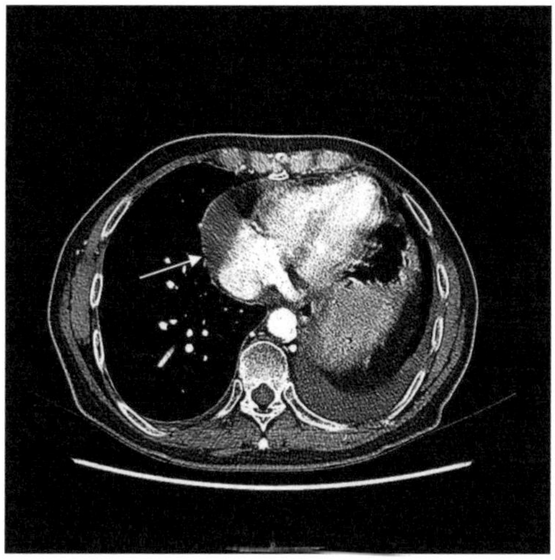

Figure 2.
Axial view of the loculated right pericardial effusion (arrow).

4. Surgical technique

4.1 Anterior thoracotomy approach

I believe for surgical approach to pericardial effusion that simple is better and the best is the enemy of the good. Like many other surgical techniques, different approaches have been described to get to the same end point. My suggested surgical approach is summarized in **Figure 3**. Left anterior thoracotomy is most commonly done in my surgical practice and it is outlined below.

As mentioned earlier, whenever possible I advocate percutaneous drainage of the pericardial effusion before bringing the patient to the operating theater. This will reduce the risk of cardiovascular collapse upon initiation of general anesthesia. Often, nonsurgical colleagues or even the patient will ask the need for surgery if the

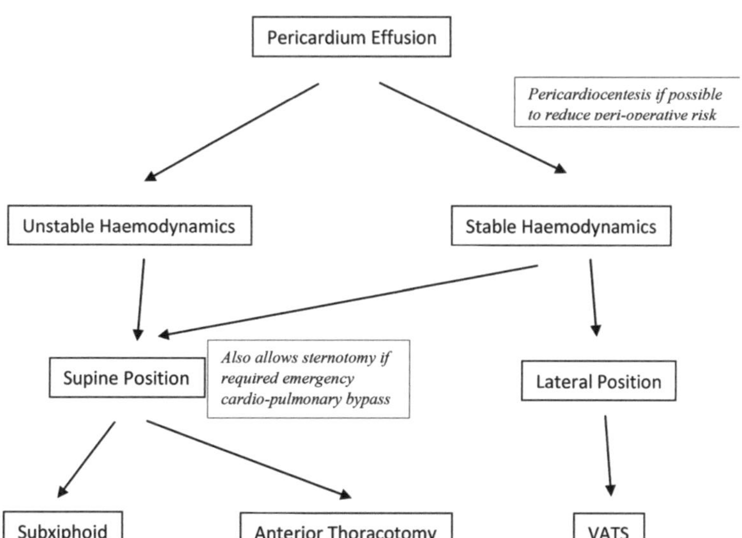

Figure 3.
Suggested flowchart for surgical approach.

effusion has been already drained. The answer is simple; creation of a surgical window is to bring about long-term benefits by reducing the risk of recurrent effusions.

The patient is positioned supine before general anesthesia via a single-lumen endotracheal tube. This approach has several advantages. Firstly, in sick and unstable patients, there is no need to turn to lateral decubitus position compared to lateral thoracotomy or VATS approaches. Conversion to midline sternotomy is also easier if required in emergency situation. Subsequently, this incision is also optimal if ascending aorta and superior vena cava cannulations are needed for crash cardiopulmonary bypass. There is always the risk of injury to the heart during surgery that requires the bypass circuit for repair. If the patient is unwell, communication with the anesthesia team is paramount. It takes an experienced anesthesiologist to intubate a patient who cannot lie flat and who requires only a little more sedation to collapse. I frequently ensure the surgical team and scrub team are ready to proceed with crash incision if required prior to onset of anesthesia.

The left anterior thoracotomy incision is made at left fourth intercostal space. This is done by surface marking the left fifth rib. I would also utilize any recent computed tomography (CT) scan of the thorax to help guide the incision over the pericardium (**Figure 4**). The incision is centered over the mid-clavicular line and extends either side to about a total of 4–5 cm in length. This is just below the nipple line in males, but care is required to avoid incision thru breast tissue in females. The incision is deepened pass the intercostal muscles, staying close and on top of the inferior fifth rib to avoid injury to any intercostal vessels. Another pitfall is to extend too medially, where the internal mammary vessels run about 1 cm from the lateral sternal margin (**Figure 4**). If done correctly, the pleural cavity is breached first, with the surface of the pericardium seen after (**Figure 5**). If the incision is too low, pericardial fat could be obscuring the actual pericardium tissue. This fat would need to be removed for adequate exposure. Further exposure could be also improved by using a sponge-stick to gently retract the lung laterally again from the pericardium.

Before incision of the pericardium, proper communication with the anesthesia team is important. Frequently, a drop in blood pressure can be encountered on drainage of the pericardial effusion. This is attributed to inadequate venous return

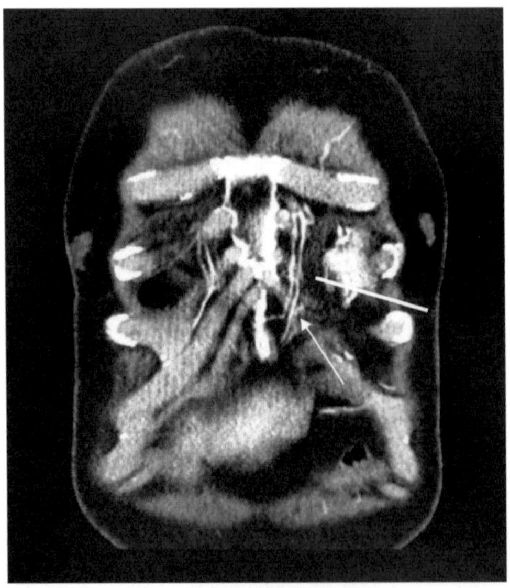

Figure 4.
CT used to plan incision at left fourth intercostal space (white line), inferior to the nipple. Take a note of the location of left internal mammary artery, about 1 cm from the lateral sternal edge (arrow).

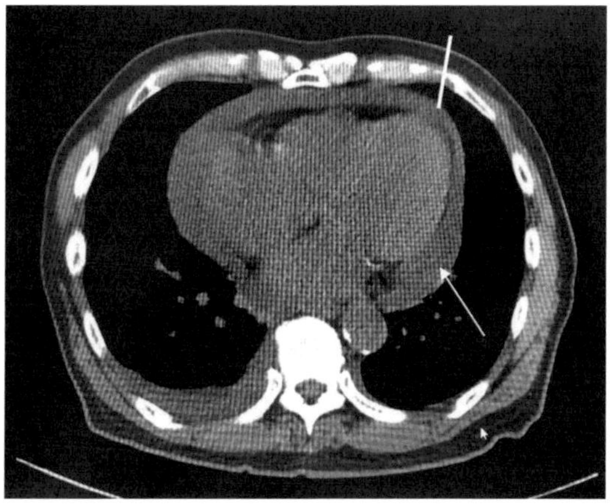

Figure 5.
Circumferential pericardial effusion (arrow) in noncontrast scan. Following the direction of the white line, left pleural cavity is breached first before the pericardium is seen.

to the patient's re-expanded heart chambers; hence, fluids should be prepared prior to drainage. Occasionally, blood-stained pericardial fluid is seen from a malignant process. If this occurs, caution is required. I suggest waiting to ensure no further hemodynamic compromise occurs before extension of the incision. Injury of the myocardium can mimic this, and even experienced surgeons can get into trouble via injury to the heart chambers.

Once the pericardial cavity is drained, I would usually excise the pericardium approximately to 3–4 cm diameter. It should be extended as laterally as possible. I believe that a bigger-sized incision and going more lateral reduces the risk of spontaneous closure of the window. A surgical pitfall is to injure the phrenic nerve which runs on the lateral pericardial surface. To avoid this, the tough pericardial tissue can be grasped and retracted towards the ceiling while the lung is retracted laterally. This is usually enough to identify the phrenic nerve and to avoid it. From this approach the pericardium can only be opened anterior to the phrenic nerve. A left-sided approach is better suited if the effusion is circumferential as minimal retraction of the lung is required to reach the pericardium (**Figure 6**). For right anterior thoracotomy, I would reserve this for redo-window creation or when there is a loculated effusion that is only accessible from the right. From the right, more of the lung is in the way before the pericardium can be seen. This may require lung isolation or even periods of intermittent apnoea from the anesthesia team for optimal visualization.

4.2 Video-assisted thoracoscopic surgery (VATS) approach

If the patient is stable enough for lung isolation via double-lumen endotracheal tube or a bronchial blocker, VATS approach can be utilized. The benefits of VATS and other minimally invasive approaches have been described at length by many authors [5, 6, 9–11]. Visualization is definitely better through a camera; the entire pericardium can be visualized once the lung is isolated well. The phrenic nerve which is the lateral limit of excision can be accurately identified and preserved. Another benefit of VATS includes a less painful incision during the perioperative period, which will reduce the amount of opioids given and hence reduces their side effects. However, this effect is less pronounced compared to my preference for the anterior thoracotomy incision, which is not that painful as there is minimal spreading of ribs. The patient could be positioned either supine or lateral position for VATS, depending on the surgeon's preference. I prefer the supine approach as

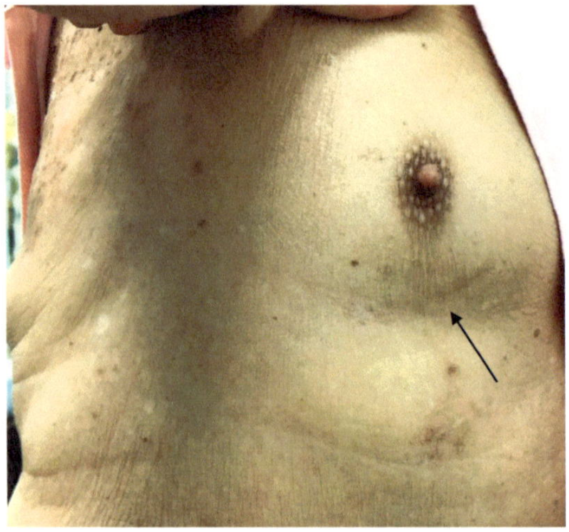

Figure 6.
Healed scar from the left anterior thoracotomy incision (arrow).

mentioned earlier; it is easier to convert to sternotomy if required. However, most surgeons would avoid sternotomy if possible, as it brings about more pain with a bigger scar as well as higher risk of infection to both the superficial tissue and sternum. The greater the surgical trauma, the longer healing requires before adjuvant treatment like chemotherapy or radiotherapy could be initiated.

4.3 Variation in anesthesia methods

Another variation of technique involves the consideration between general anesthesia and local anesthesia. General anesthesia remains the most common way of anesthesia for patients; it involves intubation and protection of airway under muscle paralysis, sedation and amnesia. But for patients who have hemodynamic compromise from pending cardiac tamponade due to a significant acute pericardial effusion, general anesthesia remains very high risk. In fact this group of patients is frequently the American Society of Anesthesiologists (ASA) class V, the highest-risk class. Many a surgeon have been demoralized after losing patients on the operating table, after this group of patients collapse upon giving the slightly amount of medication that could lower the vascular tone and reduce the blood pressures. Local anesthesia has been advocated to be safer in these patients, but often not practical as few patients could tolerate the pain of an anterior thoracotomy incision even with the best local infiltration. Mentioned later below, a subxiphoid incision could be more tolerable with this, and some surgeons have been successful with it. A new method in the middle ground could be non-intubated general anesthesia. This has been successful in reported VATS surgery [12]. Without muscle paralysis and using a laryngeal mask airway to continue spontaneous-assisted ventilation, this resulting loss of vascular tone could be reduced and perhaps reduce the risk of anesthesia. But the surgeon must also realize and cope with the increased muscle tone and continued ventilation of the lungs. Exposure needs to be ensured as the lung cannot be isolated in this setting.

4.4 Alternatives including subxiphoid approach

A subxiphoid approach (**Figure** 7) is usually less painful than VATS. The reason is that being in midline, less respiratory muscles are incised. It is also the preferred approach for patients who had recent sternotomy and subsequently presents with a

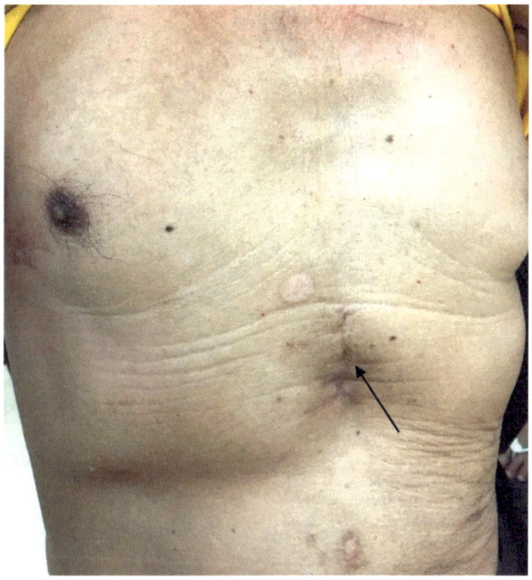

Figure 7.
Healed scar from the subxiphoid incision (arrow).

pericardial effusion. In this group of patients, rather than to redo sternotomy, only the inferior portion of the scar needs to be reopened for access to the pericardial cavity. The sternum and wires used to oppose the bone during the initial sternotomy do not require any further manipulation from this approach. This type of effusion, if related to bleeding postsurgery, usually does not recur frequently or long term; hence, this approach is simple and effective. A subxiphoid incision can be also used to create a pericardial-peritoneum window. This method, when paired with a pleuroperitoneal shunt, has been described to have comparable results to other methods [13]. The proposed shunt pumps fluid actively into the peritoneum cavity, and this can possibly reduce accumulation rates by preventing omentum from occluding the pathway from the pericardium to the peritoneum. Authors have been successful with this with only local anesthesia; hence, this alternative is useful for patients who are at high risk with general anesthesia.

5. Summary

Surgical approach to pericardial effusion involves many a thought process. Different patients require different approaches for the best results. Decision-making should be made with the patient's best interest and wishes. It is rewarding indeed when patients get symptomatic relief and are able to return to their function postsurgery.

Author details

Ing Xiang Soo
Department of Cardiothoracic Surgery, National Heart Centre Singapore, Singapore

*Address all correspondence to: soo.ing.xiang@singhealth.com.sg

IntechOpen

© 2018 The Author(s). Licensee IntechOpen. This chapter is distributed under the terms of the Creative Commons Attribution License (http://creativecommons.org/licenses/by/3.0), which permits unrestricted use, distribution, and reproduction in any medium, provided the original work is properly cited.

References

[1] Restrepo CS et al. Primary pericardial tumors. Radiographics. 2013;**33**(6):1613-1630

[2] Mayosi BM et al. Tuberculous pericarditis. Circulation. 2005;**112**:3608-3616

[3] Imazio M et al. Management of pericardial effusion. European Heart Journal. 2013;**34**:1186-1197

[4] Sasse T et al. Post-cardiac injury syndrome: Aetiology, diagnosis, and treatment. ESC E-Journal of Cardiology Practice. 2017;**15**:21-31

[5] Hurley JP et al. Video-assisted thoracic surgery for delayed pericardial effusion post-CABG. Chest. 1994;**106**(5):1617-1619

[6] O'Brien PK et al. Comparative study of subxiphoid versus video-thoracoscopic pericardial "window". The Annals of Thoracic Surgery. 2005;**80**(6):2013-2019

[7] Naunheim KS et al. Pericardial drainage: Subxiphoid vs. transthoracic approach. European Journal of Cardio-Thoracic Surgery. 1991;**5**(2):99-103

[8] Langdon SE et al. Contemporary outcomes after pericardial window surgery: Impact of operative technique. Journal of Cardiothoracic Surgery. 2016;**11**:73

[9] Sakanoue I et al. Efficacy and safety of thoracoscopic pericardial window in patients with pericardial effusions: A single-center case series. Journal of Cardiothoracic Surgery. 2016;**11**:92

[10] Muhammad MI et al. The pericardial window: Is a video-assisted thoracoscopy approach better than a surgical approach? Interactive CardioVascular and Thoracic Surgery. 2011;**12**(2):174-178

[11] Georghiou GP et al. Video-assisted thoracoscopic pericardial window for diagnosis and management of pericardial effusions. The Annals of Thoracic Surgery. 2005;**80**(2):607-610

[12] Rocco G et al. Non-intubated uniportal lung surgery. European Journal of Cardio-Thoracic Surgery. 2016;**49**:i3-i5

[13] Nan W et al. Pericardioperitoneal shunt: An alternative treatment for malignant pericardial effusion. The Annals of Thoracic Surgery. 1994;**57**:289-289

Chapter 6

Anaesthesia for Patients with Pericardial Disease

Michelle Correia

Abstract

Patients with pericardial disease can present to the anaesthesiologist for a variety of diagnostic procedures or therapeutic interventions. Providing safe anaesthesia care for these patients is challenging because of their primary pericardial pathology and significant co-morbidities affecting other organ systems. A thorough understanding of the pathophysiology of the pericardial disease state and its effect on overall haemodynamic variables is necessary before formulating a peri-operative care plan. A multidisciplinary approach involving cardiology, surgical, anaesthesia and critical care teams is needed to provide optimal peri-operative care. This chapter examines the basic pathophysiology of pericarditis, pericardial effusions, tamponade and constrictive pericarditis as these conditions pertain to the anaesthesiologist in the peri-operative period. Diagnostic tools, especially the role of echocardiography, that aid in the diagnosis and management of these high-risk patients are highlighted.

Keywords: anaesthesia, pericardial disease

1. Introduction

Patients with pericardial disease can present to the anaesthesiologist for a variety of diagnostic procedures or therapeutic interventions. Providing safe anaesthesia care for these patients is challenging because of their primary pericardial pathology and significant co-morbidities affecting other organ systems. A thorough understanding of the pathophysiology of the pericardial disease state and its effect on overall haemodynamic variables is necessary before formulating a peri-operative care plan. A multidisciplinary approach involving cardiology, surgical, anaesthesia and critical care teams is needed to provide optimal peri-operative care.

This chapter will examine the basic physical and physiological principles that govern the pathological states of pericarditis, pericardial effusion, tamponade and constrictive pericarditis. A thorough understanding of these principles is required prior to the induction of anaesthesia.

2. Normal anatomy and physiology

2.1 Normal anatomy

The normal pericardium is situated in the anterior mediastinum surrounding the heart and proximal portions of the great vessels [1–7]. It is composed of

IntechOpen

two layers: an inner visceral layer which is thin, adherent to and continuous with the epicardium of the heart and an outer parietal layer which is thicker and more fibrous. Normal pericardial thickness is 1–2 mm [8]. The parietal and visceral layers are separated by a small amount of serous fluid [1–8]. In non-disease states, approximately 15–50 ml of fluid is contained within the pericardial sac. This fluid is produced by visceral mesothelium cells and is drained from the pericardial space via the lymphatic system to the right side of the heart.

The pericardium is fixed in its anatomical position to the diaphragm and sternum via the pericardio-phrenic and sterno-pericardial ligaments, respectively [4]. Posteriorly, the loosely bound connective tissue anchors it to structures contained within the posterior mediastinum.

Vascular supply is from the pericardio-phrenic artery which is a branch of the internal thoracic artery. Venous drainage is via the pericardio-phrenic veins which drain into the brachiocephalic veins bilaterally. The phrenic nerve provides sensory innervation and the sympathetic trunks' vasomotor innervation [4].

The reflections of the pericardium surrounding the great vessels form two potential spaces called the oblique and transverse sinuses which can be visualised on echocardiographic imaging [4, 8]. The larger oblique sinus forms posteriorly between the left atrium and pulmonary veins. The transverse sinus too lies behind the left atrium, posterior to the aorta and pulmonary trunk [4]. Both sinuses are common sites for blood to collect post-cardiac surgery. Because of the formation of these two sinuses, the left atrium is not entirely an intra-pericardial structure.

2.2 Normal physiology and functions of the pericardium

Although normal cardiovascular function can occur in the absence of the pericardium, it does bestow certain physiological benefits [1–8]. Because of its relatively fixed ligamentous attachments, the pericardium stabilises the heart in its anatomic position and limits excessive movement within the chest cavity particularly with changes in body position. The pericardial fluid minimises friction exerted on the epicardium from normal heart movements during the cardiac cycle and serves to balance hydrostatic pressures over the surface of the heart. The pressure exerted on the cardiac chambers by the pressure within the intra-pericardial space prevents acute distention of the chambers and helps optimise atrial and ventricular coupling and filling. The pericardial sac serves as a physical barrier against the spread of infection or neoplastic disease within the mediastinum. Prostaglandins secreted by mesothelial and endothelial cells of the pericardium regulate autonomic cardiac reflexes, modulate myocardial contractile function and influence epicardial coronary artery tone.

3. Pathology

There are a number of pericardial pathologies which can be a cause for concern in the peri-operative period [2–4, 9, 10].

3.1 Congenital defects

Congenital defects are rare, usually associated with other cardiac, pulmonary and skeletal abnormalities, and are often only found at autopsy with an incidence of 1:10,000 [9]. The absence of the pericardium is more commonly partial with the left side being affected about 70% of the time. Left-sided defects predispose to herniation of the heart which may become haemodynamically significant during induction of anaesthesia or cause prolonged ischaemia due to compression of the coronary vessels. Right-sided defects may cause significant compression of the vena cava compromising venous return and cardiac output. Total pericardial absence is rare. Excessive cardiac motion and displacement associated with complete absence predispose to an increased risk of traumatic aortic dissection.

3.2 Acute pericarditis

Acute pericarditis is an inflammatory disease of the pericardium lasting less than 6 weeks and the most common pericardial pathology encountered in clinical practice [6, 9–16]. It may be a self-limiting benign condition or the first presentation of an underlying infectious or neoplastic disease process. In this setting, it is prudent to postpone elective surgery for diagnosis and initiation of appropriate treatment.

Causes of acute pericarditis vary widely and may be idiopathic, infectious, non-infectious or autoimmune. The most common causes encountered in the peri-operative period are non-infectious post-cardiac surgery, associated with trauma, uraemia in patients with chronic renal failure or post-myocardial infarction.

Symptoms include a sharp left precordial or retrosternal chest pain which may be pleuritic in nature and varies with posture, being decreased on sitting and increased on lying supine. The pain may radiate to the trapezius ridge. This pain referral is due to the involvement of the phrenic nerve which traverses the pericardium and supplies its sensory innervation. Often there are associated prodromal symptoms of malaise, fever and generalised myalgia. Tachycardia and tachypnoea are usually out of proportion to the low grade fever. A tri-phasic friction rub corresponding to atrial systole, ventricular systole and rapid early filling during diastole may be present on examination.

In the peri-operative period, differentiating between acute pericarditis and other causes of chest pain is of utmost importance. Careful clinical examination and special investigations should be carried out to make the correct diagnosis and allow for the institution of appropriate treatment. Three of the more important differential diagnoses are acute coronary syndrome, aortic dissection and pulmonary embolism.

Patients suffering from pericarditis associated with bacterial or fungal infections, malignancies, end-stage renal disease or post-cardiac surgery are at an increased risk to progress to pericardial effusion and tamponade [12].

Post-cardiac injury syndromes, also known as post-pericardiotomy syndromes, are being recognised as an important cause for pericardial disease [13, 14]. This clinical syndrome is characterised by a febrile illness associated with pleuritic chest pain and effusions of the pleura and pericardium. The initiating event is an injury to the pericardium, myocardium and pleura from ischaemia, post surgery or a non-iatrogenic traumatic event. In predisposed individuals, an autoimmune-mediated response is triggered that can vary from a simple, self-limiting pericarditis to a complicated pleuropericarditis, resulting in massive pericardial and pleural effusions with tamponade.

Special investigations would include a 12-lead electrocardiogram (ECG) which will show sinus tachycardia, PR interval depression and diffuse concave upward sloping ST-segment elevation. Transthoracic echocardiography (TTE) may show an associated pericardial effusion and tamponade as well as other cardiac or para-cardiac diseases.

Treatment for acute pericarditis remains symptomatic with non-steroidal anti-inflammatory drugs (NSAIDs) for pain and potentially adding colchicine as an adjunct to prevent recurrence [15]. Low-dose corticosteroids may also be introduced by the primary care team if there is an associated autoimmune disease or in the case of a post-cardiac injury syndrome [13, 14, 16].

3.3 Chronic pericarditis

Chronic pericarditis may be a result of the progression of acute disease or due to recurrent episodes of relapse [6, 9, 10]. The peri-operative management will depend on haemodynamic consequences the disease process has on patient physiological parameters.

Differentiation should be made between chronic pericarditis with ongoing inflammation, pain and fever, relapsing disease where patients have periods of being symptom free and chronic pericardial effusion with persistent fluid accumulation within the pericardial sac.

As with acute pericarditis, all elective surgery should be postponed to enable symptomatic treatment of attacks with NSAIDs, colchicine and corticosteroids. Pericardiectomy is indicated in patients with frequent and severe symptoms that are unresponsive to maximal medical therapy [6, 9].

Chronic inflammatory disease may be associated with a pericardial effusion. Moderate to large effusions, determined at echocardiography as being more than 10 mm separation of the pericardial layers during diastole, should be drained before any elective surgery takes place. Haemodynamic effects of the effusion should be assessed via echocardiographic studies and quantified prior to induction of anaesthesia as detailed below.

3.4 Pericardial effusions and tamponade

Pericardial effusion occurs when there is excessive fluid accumulation within the pericardial space [3–10, 12, 17–41]. The effusion may be transudative, exudative, haemorrhagic or purulent depending on the cause. Progressive accumulation of fluid within the pericardial sac may lead to compression of cardiac chambers, obstruction of cardiac filling and tamponade.

3.4.1 Causes for effusion

Causes of pericardial effusion are similar to those for pericarditis and may be due to the inflammatory process itself [6, 16, 18–21]. The most common causes of pericardial effusion seen in the peri-operative period are iatrogenic, associated with cardiac surgery or percutaneous coronary intervention (PCI); traumatic as seen in blunt or penetrating chest injuries; associated with malignancy; as a consequence of end-stage renal disease or dialysis; and those occurring from infectious diseases. In developing countries, especially where the prevalence of HIV is high, tuberculous pericarditis is common [6, 17].

There are a few groups of patients that require special mention as they frequently need intervention by the anaesthesiology team and present with pericardial effusions in the peri-operative period.

3.4.1.1 End-stage renal disease

Patients with end-stage renal disease (ESRD) frequently present to the anaesthesiologist for a number of diagnostic, therapeutic or vascular access procedures [6, 18–21]. The association with end-stage renal and cardiovascular disease is well established. Increased inflammatory processes, immune and autoimmune dysfunction, dyslipidaemia, endocrine abnormalities, oxidative stress and accumulation of toxic metabolites have all been suggested as causes for this association. This population is known to have an increased incidence of coronary artery disease, valvular pathology, arrhythmias and myocardial and pericardial diseases [18].

The incidence of pericarditis in ESRD is 2–21% with effusion and tamponade being present in up to 14–56% of patients. The aetiology differs between patients on haemodialysis and those who are not. Patients not yet on haemodialysis develop a uraemic pericarditis and effusions that generally respond well to aggressive dialysis and filtration. The incidence of uraemic pericarditis is decreasing because of more efficient dialyzer membranes and methods.

Patients on haemodialysis develop dialysis pericarditis with effusions that more frequently require drainage via a pericardial window procedure. This group of patients has a higher incidence of progressing to constrictive pericarditis possibly requiring pericardiectomy [18]. Progression from effusion to tamponade may be difficult to diagnose, but progressive right heart failure and hypotension in the setting of adequate diuresis is highly suggestive [18]. All patients with ESRD presenting for surgery should have pre-operative investigations to rule out significant pericardial disease that may impact on peri-operative management.

Indications for drainage of effusions in these patients are based on clinical and biochemical features. Dialysis pericarditis, tachypnoea >20 breaths/min, fever >39°C, low voltage complexes on 12-lead ECG, hypoalbuminaemia <31 g/l, leukocytosis and any signs of tamponade on TTE all indicate the need for drainage [18]. There are little data to support one drainage procedure over another [6, 18]. Pericardiocentesis and pericardial window are both acceptable methods for relief of raised intra-pericardial pressure.

Although these patients may exhibit signs of large effusions and even tamponade, significant haemodynamic compromise associated with anaesthesia is rare in this group of patients. Because of the chronicity of the disease process and the associated hypertension, careful titration of agents used for general anaesthesia to facilitate drainage procedures is usually well tolerated [21].

3.4.1.2 Post-cardiac surgery and post-operative pericardial effusions (PPE)

Patients post-cardiac surgery are another group whose management frequently requires the involvement of the anaesthesiology team [24, 32–38]. Accumulation of blood within the pericardial sac because of ongoing bleeding from either a surgical or medical cause peri-operatively will lead to the development of PPE and tamponade. PPE can be divided into early, presenting within 7 days, and late complications occurring more than 7 days post-procedure. An important cause of persistent PPE is the inflammatory response associated with post-cardiac injury syndrome [13, 14, 33].

The incidence for PPE has a wide range depending on the study quoted and is approximately 20% on the 20th post-operative day [33]. Most effusions are clinically insignificant, defined as less than 10 mm in diastole on TTE, and resolve spontaneously after reaching their maximum volume on day 10 post-operatively [33]. The incidence of significant pre-tamponade and tamponade requiring re-intervention is 1–2.6% [33].

Presenting symptoms are usually non-specific consisting of tachycardia, hypotension, tachypnoea, orthopnoea and decreased heart sounds [24, 32–34]. This low cardiac output state must be differentiated from other common causes of cardiogenic shock in the post-operative period. The differential diagnosis would include hypovolaemia, significant ischaemia, ventricular dysfunction or severe inflammatory response syndrome [32].

The following have been identified as independent risk factors for the development of post-operative effusions [33, 34, 37]: heart transplantation, pulmonary thromboembolism, aortic aneurysm surgery, increased body surface area, valve surgery, immunosuppression, urgent or emergent surgery, renal failure and prolonged cardiopulmonary bypass (CPB) times. In other studies, female gender, pre-operative use of anticoagulants and early chest drain removal have been associated with increased incidence of PPE [33, 37].

In the setting of post-operative haemodynamic deterioration, critical tamponade may develop quickly with even small amounts of fluid accumulation causing significant haemodynamic effects. The diagnosis should be made immediately in order to facilitate life-saving intervention. TTE remains the diagnostic tool of choice because it is non-invasive and has a high sensitivity and specificity for detecting the signs of cardiac tamponade [6, 24, 32, 35, 38]. It may also be useful in confirming or ruling out other causes for post-operative haemodynamic deterioration. Because tamponade is a dynamic pathological process, especially in the post-operative period, serial or repeat echocardiographic examinations coupled with ongoing clinical evaluation are necessary to ensure appropriate and timeous management.

Although TTE remains the diagnostic tool of choice, detecting effusions and tamponade post-operatively may be challenging [31, 32, 38]. Patients who have altered anatomy are most likely to be on positive pressure ventilation with positive end expiratory pressure (PEEP), may have pneumopericardium (air trapped in the pericardium) and will have drains in situ. Effusions post cardiac surgery are often loculated causing regional compression of only one or some of the cardiac chambers. Blood and clots collect in the posterior sinuses making diagnosis via the traditionally accepted criteria on TTE difficult. Trans-oesophageal echocardiography (TOE) is well tolerated in sedated or anaesthetised patients but is more invasive and may not be readily available. Supplemental modalities such as CT scan and cardiac MRI have been suggested to aid in the diagnosis when TTE is inconclusive [6, 31, 38].

Indications for drainage of effusions are based on clinical and TTE findings of tamponade: left ventricular dysfunction in patients receiving intermittent positive pressure ventilation, loculated effusions or clots causing compression of the left atrium or left ventricle, documented collapse of right-sided chambers and if pericardial separation is >20 mm [3, 32, 35].

Anaesthetic management of post-operative effusions and tamponade remains the same as for an effusion from any other cause. The need for ongoing inotropic support and appropriate mechanical ventilation, massive fluid shifts, ongoing bleeding due to surgical causes, coagulopathy due to anticoagulant use, intrinsic clotting abnormalities, need for massive blood transfusion, renal dysfunction and the significant risks of re-sternotomy are just a few of the unique challenges for the anaesthesiologist to consider when taking a cardiac patient back to theatre for re-intervention. Drainage procedures are most often limited to pericardiocentesis under ultrasound- or video-assisted guidance [25, 32, 35]. A small percentage of patients may require sternotomy for the effective management of post-operative effusions [25, 32].

3.4.1.3 Effusions in patients undergoing percutaneous cardiac interventions

Percutaneous intracardiac intervention is a risk factor for the development of pericardial effusion and tamponade [39–41]. The exact incidence depends on the procedure performed, the extent of the intervention, whether it is diagnostic or therapeutic, and if anticoagulation is used in the peri-procedural period. The exact procedure-specific incidence is difficult to determine, and small to moderate effusions may occur much more frequently than studies suggest [39]. The incidence of tamponade ranges from <1 to 6% depending on the study being quoted. Some of the more commonly performed interventions include atrial fibrillation ablation associated with a 4% risk of tamponade, permanent pacemaker insertion which carries a 1.7% risk of cardiac perforation and life-threatening tamponade and left atrial appendage (LAA) occlusion procedures which are associated with a 1.8–3% risk of tamponade, most commonly due to LAA perforation.

The overall incidence of tamponade following percutaneous coronary intervention (PCI) is 0.12% and is associated with high mortality [40, 41]. Coronary artery perforation following percutaneous coronary intervention is found in 0.3% of patients of which 10% went on to develop tamponade [41]. The risks were increased in patients requiring more complex interventions and if athero-ablative procedures were performed instead of angioplasty and stent placement.

Pericardial effusion and tamponade following PCI usually present acutely in the catheterisation lab but can have an insidious onset and are an important cause for late hypotension post intervention [40].

The diagnosis of tamponade post PCI remains predominately clinical and should be confirmed with TTE and other imaging techniques as soon as possible in order to facilitate life-saving treatment drainage procedures as described below.

3.4.2 Pathophysiology of pericardial effusions

The haemodynamic effects of the effusion and the development of tamponade are dependent on the rate of fluid accumulation within the pericardial space, the total volume of fluid that accumulates, the type of the fluid that accumulates and the intrinsic compliance of the pericardial tissue layers [4, 5, 7, 24].

Because the pericardium is relatively stiff, it has a limited reserve volume. Small but rapidly accumulating effusions quickly exceed the compliance of the parietal layer. Once the limit of pericardial stretch is exceeded, even small increases in volume cause a steep increase in pericardial pressure causing external compression of the cardiac chambers and tamponade.

Chronic accumulation over a prolonged period allows for pericardial stretch and compensatory mechanisms meaning that the intra-pericardial pressure remains low despite a large amount of fluid within the space. Even with additive amounts of fluid, the pericardial compliance curve remains less steep than in the acute setting resulting in slower increases in intra-pericardial pressures relative to the volume of fluid within the space.

The type of fluid that accumulates may influence the haemodynamic presentation. Exudative fluid may become fibrinous and cause constriction, haemorrhagic fluid may contain clots causing isolated chamber compression and chronic effusions may become fibrotic and confining.

The compliance of the pericardial tissues is also an important determining factor in the overall haemodynamic effects of an effusion. Pericardial compliance is decreased in mesothelioma, scarring from previous cardiac surgery and constrictive states.

Once intra-pericardial and intracardiac pressures increase beyond a certain limit, cardiac chamber filling and preload are reduced which causes a drop in stroke volume and cardiac output. This decrease in cardiac output causes a reduction in organ perfusion which triggers compensatory mechanisms including activation of the sympathetic nervous system and the renin-angiotensin-aldosterone axis. The resultant tachycardia, peripheral vasoconstriction and fluid retention are an attempt to maintain systemic blood pressure and organ perfusion in the face of a low cardiac output state.

3.5 Tamponade

Tamponade physiology occurs when cardiac chambers exhibit compression due to an increase in intra-pericardial pressures and equalisation of transmural pressures [3–10, 14–17, 22–24].

3.5.1 Causes of tamponade

Patients most at risk for the development of tamponade are those with iatrogenic causes post-cardiac surgery, PCI, insertion of pacemaker or percutaneous valve repair, chest trauma where blunt injuries are five times more commonly associated with tamponade when compared with penetrating injuries [25], malignant disease which is the most common cause of cardiac tamponade accounting for up to 60% of cases [25] and ESRD. Uraemic disease accounts for 10–15% of cases, while the incidence of dialysis pericarditis is 12% in patients on long-term haemodialysis [18–21].

3.5.2 Pathophysiology of cardiac tamponade

Under normal circumstances, intra-pericardial pressures reflect intrathoracic pressures and are negative [3–10, 12, 21–31]. As fluid accumulates within the pericardial space, the intra-pericardial pressures increase. Pericardial pressures are elevated throughout the cardiac cycle and cause compression of chambers for the duration of diastole when intracardiac chamber pressures are lowest.

Impaired filling of the cardiac chambers leads to diastolic dysfunction and a type of obstructive shock [23]. The venous return pattern to the atria eventually becomes unimodal and is confined to ventricular systole. In severe tamponade, atrial filling only occurs when ventricular contraction forces the atrioventricular valvular apparatus towards the myocardial apex. This caudad motion of the tricuspid and mitral valves causes a decrease in atrial pressures and enhanced systemic and pulmonary venous return.

As tamponade physiology progresses, ventricular filling becomes highly dependent on atrial systole as the intra-pericardial pressures increase. The maintenance of a sinus cardiac rhythm becomes paramount to ensure adequate ventricular filling to maintain end-diastolic ventricular volumes which are equivalent to ventricular stroke volume.

Physiologically speaking, cardiac chamber filling pressures are dependent on the myocardial transmural pressure gradient expressed mathematically by the following:

$$\text{transmural pressure} = \text{intra-pericardial pressure} - \text{intracardiac pressure}$$

The intracardiac pressures are different for each chamber with right atrial pressures being the lowest to facilitate systemic venous return.

Based on Ohm's law (V = IR), in order to ensure filling and forward flow in a normal series circulation, there must be a pressure gradient (P1–P2 or V) between the systemic venous return and the aorta. The pressure gradients below are often seen during diagnostic cardiac catheterisation procedures when venous and arterial pressures are obtained and documented:

systemic venous return pressure ➢ right atrial pressure ➢ right ventricular end-diastolic pressure ➢ right ventricular systolic pressure ➢ pulmonary capillary wedge pressure ➢ pulmonary venous return pressure ➢ left atrial pressure ➢ left ventricular end-diastolic pressure ➢ left ventricular systolic pressure ➢ aorta

As the intra-pericardial pressure increases, extrinsic compression of the cardiac chambers occurs. Compression causes the intracardiac chamber pressures to increase, and the transmural pressures begin to equalise. Right-sided filling pressures during diastole are lower than the left and are the first to be equalled and then exceeded by the increasing intra-pericardial pressures.

The right atrium and ventricle are compressed, right-sided chamber filling is compromised and the right atrial pressure, measured clinically as the central venous pressure (CVP), increases to try and maintain right ventricular filling. This causes a significant decrease in the venous return to the right heart as right atrial pressures exceed systemic venous return pressures.

A decrease in right atrial venous return leads to impaired right ventricular filling, an underloaded right ventricle which functions at the lower end of the Frank-Starling curve and a resultant decrease in right ventricular stroke volume. Reductions in right ventricular stroke volume translate into decreased flow through the pulmonary circulation with decreased pulmonary venous return to the left atrium. With continued increases in the intra-pericardial pressures, equalisation of left-sided pressures eventually transpires. This results in massive reductions in and eventual cessation of diastolic filling and forward flow of blood through the heart with dramatically reduced cardiac output.

A cycle of exhaustive physiological compensation follows with eventual cardiac arrest manifested as pulseless electrical activity. Although reductions in coronary blood flow do occur with the drop in cardiac output and aortic diastolic pressures, this is coupled with limited cardiac work, and ischaemia is usually avoided.

It is of utmost importance to note that the equalisation of transmural pressures found in cardiac tamponade is a dynamic process influenced by extra-cardiac factors. Induction of general anaesthesia causes a decrease in heart rate, vasodilation and direct myocardial depression. Coupled with the institution of positive pressure ventilation, massive decreases in venous return and cardiac output occur. Thus, induction of anaesthesia may precipitate complete cardiovascular collapse in patients with tamponade.

Patients at risk for the development of tamponade should therefore have echocardiographic studies to confirm their pre-operative haemodynamic state. In the event of potential or imminent tamponade, all elective procedures should be postponed and the pericardium drained via the most appropriate method to relieve transmural pressures before induction of anaesthesia is performed.

3.5.3 Classification of tamponade

Not all cases of cardiac tamponade are uniform, and patients can present with different forms [24, 25].

Low-pressure tamponade occurs at very low diastolic pressures of 6–12 mmHg and is present in patients with severe hypovolaemia. Patients do not present with the full clinical picture of tamponade until they have been adequately fluid resuscitated and are fluid replete. This form is often found in trauma patients with ongoing haemorrhage or post-cardiac surgery.

Regional tamponade occurs when only specific cardiac chambers are compressed from localised amassing of fluid. This is a common finding post-cardiac surgery or myocardial infarction. Typical clinical findings of acute tamponade are often absent necessitating multimodal diagnostic imaging to make the diagnosis.

Hypertensive tamponade is said to be present when there are classical features of tamponade but with elevated arterial pressures, sometimes over 200 mmHg. It is thought to be due to excessive beta-adrenergic drive in patients with pre-existing hypertension.

Effusive-constrictive pericarditis is present when there is decreased pericardial compliance with a reduced pericardial cavity associated with an effusion. Constrictive physiology is present, and tamponade can occur even with minimal amounts of fluid accumulation. A variety of haemodynamic and imaging signs make for a mixed clinical picture. Drainage of the effusive fluid provides the best clue as symptoms of constriction persist in spite of appropriate drainage.

3.5.3.1 Clinical signs and diagnosis

Dyspnoea, orthopnoea, diaphoresis, chest pain and tachycardia are all non-specific signs of pericardial effusion and tamponade. Muffled heart sounds, raised jugular venous pressure and hypotension are the features classically described as Beck's triad used in the diagnosis.

Pulsus paradoxus is a clinical sign commonly found in tamponade and refers to the exaggeration of the normal physiological variation in systolic blood pressure of more than 10 mmHg during negative pressure ventilation. Under normal physiological conditions, the intra-pericardial pressure mirrors intrathoracic pressures. Negative intrathoracic pressure generated on inspiration is transmitted to the heart, and the intra-pericardial pressure decreases. This in turn increases the transmural pressure gradient. The increase in transmural pressure gradient augments right atrial and ventricular filling during diastole. This is demonstrated on Doppler echocardiography by increased blood flow velocity across the tricuspid valve during inspiration [28].

The augmentation in right ventricular filling causes the intra-ventricular septum to shift to the left which transiently impacts on left ventricular filling. This is known as *interventricular dependence.* With normal pericardial pressures and compliance, compensation for this slight shift is maintained leading to minimal reductions in left ventricular end-diastolic volume. There is a small decrease in left ventricular stroke volume and cardiac output which results in a small decrease in systolic blood pressure during inspiration of not more than 10 mmHg. The augmented right ventricular stroke volume during inspiration translates into increased pulmonary venous return to the left atrium after several cardiac cycles. An increase in left ventricular stroke volume and systolic blood pressure is then seen during expiration.

In cardiac tamponade, this normal systolic pressure variation with respiration is exaggerated. With the decrease in pericardial compliance, the normal pericardial compensation for the left heart shift is lost. As the intra-ventricular septum shifts to the left, the left heart cannot expand because of the increased intra-pericardial pressures. Left ventricular filling and flow through the left ventricular outflow tract are affected to a greater degree resulting in *enhanced ventricular interdependence.* This translates into a decrease of systolic blood pressure of more than 10 mmHg during inspiration.

Pulsus paradoxus is not very sensitive or specific for cardiac tamponade and may be absent even when tamponade is present or be present with conditions other than tamponade [22, 24, 25].

Pulsus may be absent in the presence of tamponade with severe aortic regurgitation where left ventricular filling is maintained due to back flow from the aorta; with localised effusions or clot that compress only certain chambers of the heart; with an atrial septal defect where the pressure effect on the right atrium is balanced by the intra-cardiac shunt; and with severe right ventricular hypertrophy with pulmonary hypertension where the pressure effects from increased intra-pericardial pressure on right heart are less pronounced.

Pulsus paradoxus may exist in the absence of tamponade in severe chronic obstructive pulmonary disease, asthma or severe bronchospasm, hypovolaemia, congestive cardiac failure and obesity.

Pulsus paradoxus will be reversed in patients receiving *positive pressure ventilation* with increased systolic blood pressure noted on inspiration and a fall in systolic blood pressure on expiration [22, 25]. This can be interpreted as systolic pressure variation in patients receiving mechanical ventilation which is often used clinically as a sign of fluid responsiveness.

Mechanical ventilation with PEEP has three main effects on cardiac physiology. (1) With the increase in intra-thoracic pressure, alveolar pressures increase more than pleural pressures which causes compression of pulmonary capillaries and increased right ventricular afterload. (2) Compression of pulmonary capillaries squeezes blood from the pulmonary bed into the left atrium augmenting left ventricular preload. (3) Positive inspiratory pressure augments left ventricular systolic function.

The augmentation of left ventricular stroke volume and systolic function during inspiration leads to increased systolic blood pressures. Pulmonary transit time is approximately 2 s, and the drop in right heart cardiac output from positive intrathoracic pressures translates into a drop in left ventricular cardiac output and systolic blood pressure during expiration. A reversed pattern of pulsus paradoxus is seen.

As mentioned above, the combination of decreased venous return or preload to the right heart with induction of anaesthesia plus the increased right ventricular afterload effects of mechanical ventilation can severely compromise cardiac function in patients with tamponade.

3.5.3.2 Special investigations

Chest X-ray will show an enlarged globular bottle-shaped cardiac shadow if the pericardial fluid volume is >200 ml, a widened mediastinum with a right costophrenic angle <90° and clear lung fluids [7–10, 12, 21–29]. There may be an associated pleural effusion that requires concurrent drainage and management.

ECG may show a sinus tachycardia which is the most common finding. Other findings may include low QRS and T wave voltages, PR segment depression, nonspecific ST-T wave changes and bundle branch block. Electrical alternans is the change in QRS voltage with each beat and reflects excessive swinging movement of the heart within a large effusion [21].

TTE is the investigation of choice to diagnose and evaluate pericardial disease [3–6, 12, 23–28, 30, 31]. It is a class 1 recommendation with a high sensitivity and specificity for the detection of effusions and tamponade. TTE in addition allows for the evaluation of myocardial and endocardial structures and function, aiding to rule out other causes for the clinical picture. A grading system for the size of the effusion is based on echo-free space in diastole with small effusions being <10 mm in size, moderate effusions 10–20 mm and large effusions >20 mm. Right atrial collapse and invagination for >30% of the cardiac cycle on ECHO is 100% sensitive for the diagnosis of tamponade [26].

Other TTE signs of tamponade include distention and loss of respiratory variation in the size of the IVC which reflects increased right atrial pressures, increased respiratory variations in tricuspid and mitral trans-valvular inflow velocities on Doppler studies, intra-ventricular septal shift reflected clinically as pulsus paradoxus [26], localised or loculated effusions showing isolated chamber compression and regional tamponade commonly encountered post-cardiac surgery [32].

Cardiac catheterisation is usually not performed in acute tamponade as TTE is less invasive, less time-consuming and diagnostic. If catheterisation is performed, a blunted Y descent may be demonstrated [29]. The Y descent on the CVP tracing after the v wave indicates opening of the tricuspid valve and reflects early diastolic filling of the right ventricle. Attenuation of the y descent reflects rapid equalisation of pressures between the right atrium and ventricle which leads to ineffective ventricular filling during early diastole in tamponade (**Figure 1**).

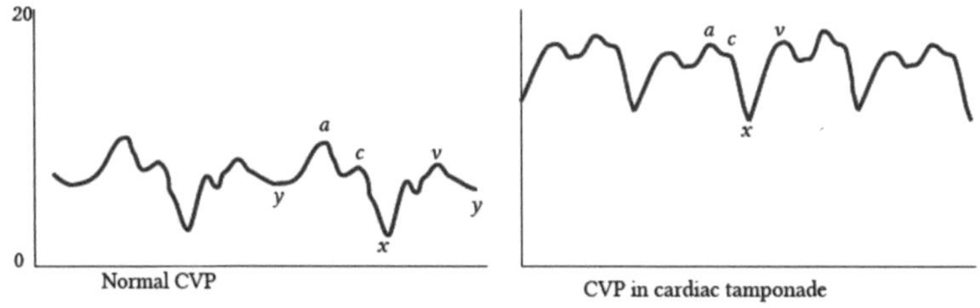

Figure 1.
CVP tracing in cardiac tamponade reflecting higher baseline pressures and attenuation of the y descent.

3.5.4 Medical management of pericardial effusions and tamponade

In about 60% of cases of pericardial effusion, an underlying disease process is known, and medical management would therefore be targeted at the aetiology [6]. In the absence of significant associated inflammation, NSAIDs, colchicine and steroids are generally ineffective, leaving no conservative management options for isolated effusions. In these instances, surgical drainage is indicated.

3.6 Constrictive pericarditis (CP)

Chronic inflammation of the pericardium causes it to thicken and become non-compliant and rigid [4, 6, 7, 9, 10, 12, 25, 31, 43–49]. This thickening may be concentric or regional depending on the cause. The pericardial space becomes obliterated as the visceral and parietal layers change and stiffen. Restriction of cardiac chamber expansion during diastole causes impedance of cardiac filling and diastolic dysfunction at both the atrial and ventricular levels. The usual form is constriction without effusion but effusive-constrictive forms can occur.

3.6.1 Causes of constrictive pericarditis

Causes are similar to those for acute and chronic pericarditis including infectious disease, radiation to the mediastinum, trauma and autoimmune conditions [4, 13, 14, 48, 49]. In the developing world, tuberculosis remains the most common cause with a prevalence of >90% in places where the HIV infection rates are high [49].

Post-cardiac surgery is the most common cause of CP in the peri-operative period. The usual presentation is constrictive pathophysiology with an increase in pericardial membrane thickness. However, constrictive pathophysiology may present in the absence of pericardial membrane thickening [4, 48].

Post surgery, blood in the pericardial space causes a post-pericardiotomy-type picture with inflammation and adhesions [4, 13, 14]. These adhesions diminish the pericardial space and cause a constrictive pathophysiological picture in spite of normal pericardial thickness. This is termed *normal thickness constrictive pericarditis*. In a Mayo Clinic study from 2003, 18% of patients with proven constriction who underwent pericardiectomy had a normal pericardial thickness of <2 mm on pre-operative imaging [48]. Disease of the pericardium in the normal thickness group consisted of mild focal areas of inflammation, calcification and fibrosis. The majority of patients were post-cardiac surgery and post chest irradiation or had suffered previous infective or idiopathic disease. Pericardiectomy was equally effective in relieving the disease symptoms in these patients compared with those who had a pericardial thickness > 2 mm. It would therefore seem reasonable to consider pericardiectomy in patients with a normal pericardial thickness if the endocardial biopsy is negative for restrictive cardiomyopathy [4, 48].

3.6.2 Pathophysiology of CP

Under normal circumstances, the pericardium can accommodate changes in cardiac volume [4, 6, 9, 12, 25, 43, 46, 47, 49]. With ongoing inflammation, the pericardial compliance decreases. The now thickened, calcified and rigid pericardium encases the heart and limits cardiac chamber expansion during diastole. Initially, early diastolic filling is not affected, and the atrial contribution to ventricular filling is mostly impeded during mid- to late diastole.

Over time, diastolic filling becomes severely impaired, and the total blood volume within the heart remains relatively constant during diastole, leading to a *fixed stroke volume state*. Any increases in tissue perfusion demands must therefore be met by an increase in heart rate.

One of the most important features of CP is that changes in intrathoracic pressures during the respiratory cycle are *not transmitted to the heart*. This is because the pericardial space has been destroyed by the inflammatory process and intrapericardial pressure no longer mirrors intrathoracic pressures [25]. This means that the normal augmentation of venous return to the right heart during inspiration does not occur. Lack of inspiratory decline in the jugular venous pressure leads rather to an increase in CVP with inspiration which is known as Kussmaul's sign.

Respiratory variation in systolic blood pressures may still be seen clinically as the pulmonary veins lie outside of the pericardium and the left atrium is only partially within the pericardial sac. Changes in intrathoracic pressures will therefore still cause changes in pulmonary vein flow despite the uncoupling of intra-pericardial and intrathoracic pressures [4]. During negative pressure ventilation, inspiration will cause the pressure gradient between the pulmonary veins and the left ventricle to decrease, resulting in a decrease in LV filling and a small decrease in systolic blood pressure. This effect, however, is not enough to cause pulsus paradoxus.

Another important pathophysiological feature of CP is the dramatic increase in ventricular interdependence [45]. Pressure changes in one ventricle will be transferred to the other which explains the observed equilibration of diastolic ventricular pressures. This increase in ventricular coupling means that there is little, if any, trans-septal pressure gradient during diastole. Abnormal shifting of the intraventricular septum has been observed in some studies but because the ventricles are operating at much higher baseline diastolic pressures, small changes in pressures caused by septal shift have very little effect on overall ventricular filling.

Chronic constriction of the myocardium can lead to damage of the underlying muscle tissue. Constriction causes the ventricles to operate at the lower end of the Frank-Starling curve which causes a kind of disuse atrophy within the myocardium. Myocardial atrophy may present with continued diastolic dysfunction coupled with significant systolic dysfunction even after successful pericardiectomy is performed and the myocardium is released. Often these patients will require ongoing inotropic support in the peri-operative setting.

3.6.2.1 Clinical signs and diagnosis

Signs and symptoms are usually non-specific and mimic right ventricular failure making diagnosis difficult [4, 6, 12, 25]. Tachycardia is the predominant sign because of the fixed stroke volume state. Arrhythmias, especially atrial fibrillation, are not uncommon. Fluid overload ranging from peripheral oedema to anasarca is a usual finding. This is due to venous hypertension which is often worsened by protein-losing enteropathy in decompensated disease. Patients may have associated pleural effusions and cachexia, indicating a chronic and insidious disease process.

Decreased cardiac output with shortness of breath and fatiguability are almost always elicited on thorough enquiry. Ascites, hepatomegaly, pleural effusion and peripheral oedema can be misdiagnosed as chronic liver disease.

Classical clinical findings in CP include a pericardial knock and Kussmaul's sign. A pericardial knock is a high-pitched sound occurring in early diastole before the third heart sound. It indicates the cessation of ventricular filling at the end of the early diastole due to the pericardial constriction.

Kussmaul's sign is a paradoxical increase in jugular venous pressure on inspiration. It reflects an increase in right atrial preload from an increase in intra-abdominal pressure during inspiration. This increased venous return from the intra-abdominal veins is independent of intrathoracic pressure changes. The increase in preload cannot be accommodated because of the fixed pericardial constriction, and the back pressure is transmitted to the systemic venous system. This is detected clinically as increased pressure in the jugular vein.

The differential diagnosis for constrictive pericarditis is important to consider as clinical signs can be confusing. Restrictive cardiomyopathy, pulmonary embolus, right ventricular infarction, pleural effusion and chronic obstructive pulmonary disease can all have a similar clinical presentation.

3.6.2.2 Special investigations

The diagnosis of constrictive pericarditis remains challenging, and the clinical picture of unexplained venous congestion should be clarified with multiple imaging modalities to ensure accurate and efficient diagnosis [4, 6, 12, 25, 31].

Chest X-ray may show a ring of calcification around the heart and cardiomegaly if there is an associated effusion.

ECG may show low voltages, non-specific upward sloping ST-T wave changes, atrial fibrillation and P mitrale, indicating chronic atrial hypertension.

CT scan and MRI are both useful to confirm pericardial thickening and calcification [4, 31]. CT scan can delineate and quantify the degree of calcification based on CT scan score, and MRI has a 93% accuracy for differentiating CP from restrictive cardiomyopathy based on a pericardial thickness of >4 mm.

TOE has a high sensitivity for the detection of features consistent with the diagnosis [12]. An increase in pericardial thickness > 2 mm, abrupt inspiratory posterior motion of the intra-ventricular septum in diastole and a non-pulsatile dilated IVC indicating venous hypertension are all expected echocardiographic features.

Pulsed wave Doppler on echocardiography can be used to assess the mitral trans-valvular inflow velocity pattern. Classically, an increase in the E wave velocity represents rapid early diastolic filling. Significant reductions in the A wave velocity represents decreased flow in mid- to late diastole. This indicates rapid early filling with premature equalisation of left atrial and left ventricular pressures from pericardial constriction.

Reverse pulmonary vein flow changes will be detectable as the poor left atrial compliance and raised left atrial pressures redirect flow back into the pulmonary veins. This results in decreased left atrial filling and decreased left ventricular end-diastolic volume.

Cardiac catheterisation may reveal a classical square root sign pattern on the right ventricular trace. This is because right ventricular pressures drop rapidly in early diastole which causes a "dip" in the trace as a small amount of blood enters the right ventricle. The limit of RV distensibility is quickly reached because of constriction by the rigid pericardium. Rapid equalisation of right atrial, right ventricular and pulmonary wedge pressures occurs, and blood flow across the tricuspid valve ceases abruptly causing a "plateau" in the pressure tracing (**Figure 2**).

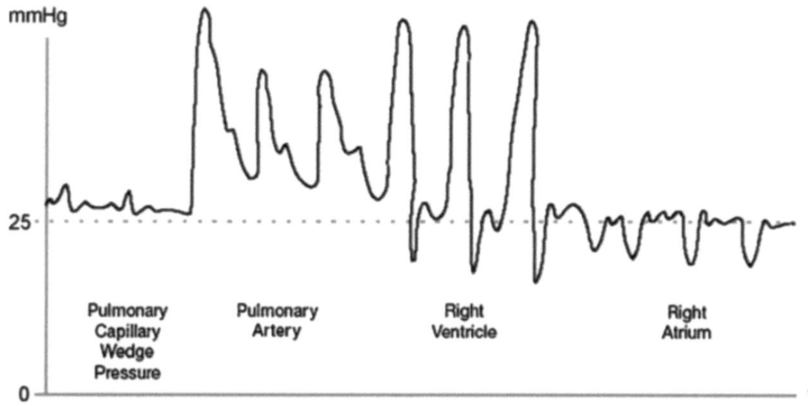

Figure 2.
Right ventricular pressure tracings: pulmonary capillary wedge pressure, pulmonary artery pressure, right ventricular pressure and right atrial pressure with diastolic equalisation of pressures and sharp "y-dip" in the case of CP [46].

Kussmaul and Vaitkus were the first to delineate criteria for correctly diagnosing CP in patients on whom cardiac catheterisations were performed. They identified three criteria that could be used in the diagnosis: a left and right ventricular end-diastolic pressure difference of <5 mmHg, a ratio of right ventricular end-diastolic pressures to right ventricular systolic pressures of >1.3 and a right ventricular systolic pressure of <50 mmHg. If all three criteria are present and patients have clinical features in keeping with the condition, CP will be correctly diagnosed in >90% of patients [49].

3.6.3 Medical management for constrictive pericarditis

Medical management is focused on the underlying cause of the pathology and may include diuretics, digoxin and beta-blockers to decrease venous congestion and tachyarrhythmias pre-operatively [9, 12, 46, 47, 49]. In the cases of TB pericarditis, anti-tuberculous chemotherapeutic treatment is required for a minimum of 2 months before surgery but can be continued for up to 12 months pre-operatively.

3.6.4 Differentiating constrictive pericarditis (CP) from restrictive cardiomyopathy (RC)

Many of the features of CP can also be found in RC making the diagnosis difficult [4, 6, 9, 12]. Restrictive cardiomyopathy is an intrinsic myocardial disease resulting in impaired relaxation and reduced compliance of cardiac chambers with severe diastolic dysfunction and atrial hypertension. Causes include infiltrative disorders such as amyloidosis, haemosiderosis and sarcoidosis or endomyocardial fibroelastosis found in scleroderma, radiotherapy or idiopathic disease.

The most important differentiating features in CP are the uncoupling of intrathoracic and intracardiac pressures and the increased ventricular interdependence. In RC, normal respiratory variation will be found on the CVP tracing. Conduction defects are also more common in patients with RC.

Differentiating features can also be elicited on TTE investigation [12]. E wave velocities reflecting early diastolic filling are reduced in RC because the intrinsic myocardial disease affects ventricular filling throughout the whole of diastole. Transmitral inflow velocity variation and respiratory variation in pulmonary vein flows are rarely found in RC. Atrial enlargement is marked reflecting severe atrial hypertension. Left ventricular hypertrophy is a common finding, and pericardial thickness will be normal. Pericardial calcifications will be absent in RC.

4. Anaesthetic management

4.1 Pericardial effusions and tamponade

4.1.1 Pre-operatively

Accumulation of fluid in the pericardial space is the primary problem, and therefore definitive drainage and relief of the raised intra-pericardial pressure are required [9, 12, 21, 22, 32]. The type of drainage procedure will depend on the aetiology of the pericardial effusion and the clinical condition of the patient. A multidisciplinary team approach is needed, and a thorough pre-operative workup should be done if time allows. Clinical history and examination should be carried out focusing on pertinent physiological symptoms and signs to identify the cause and severity of the pathology.

Patients fall broadly into two categories: pericardial effusion with pre-tamponade physiology and a haemodynamically stable clinical picture or features of tamponade are present on TTE with haemodynamic consequences and instability. The presence of orthopnoea and pulsus paradoxus is a sign of a severely compromised patient.

If there is haemodynamic compromise, the safest and quickest drainage option needs to be selected. Haemodynamic goals pre-drainage should follow the "Airway, Breathing, Circulation" approach bearing in mind the pathophysiology of tamponade as discussed above. If required, a definitive airway management strategy should be employed and supplemental oxygen administered in order to optimise the delivery of oxygen to tissues during the decreased cardiac output state. Positive pressure ventilation should be avoided, but if required, peak airway pressures and PEEP should be minimised to avoid precipitation of cardiovascular collapse.

Large-bore peripheral access is needed for fluid and blood product administration and should be secured before any pharmacological agents are administered. Invasive arterial and central venous lines are needed for monitoring but should not delay drainage for patients in extremis.

Optimisation of preload is advised pre-operatively as hypovolaemia will worsen tamponade physiology. Dynamic measures of fluid responsiveness should be used to guide fluid therapy. A single, individualised fluid challenge may be beneficial, and outcome-based measures should be used to assess response. Improvement will be if the patient reports relief of symptoms or markers of end-organ perfusion improve.

Caution needs to be exercised as too much fluid will worsen the ventricular interdependence and further compromise cardiac output. Volume loading pre-drainage may also exacerbate volume overload post-drainage. Temporary haemodynamic support with a vasopressor agent may be more appropriate than excessive fluid administration to maintain blood pressure in the pre-operative period.

4.1.2 Types of drainage procedures

Needle pericardiocentesis consists of percutaneous placement of a catheter into the pericardial sac to facilitate external drainage of the effusion [24, 25]. Specific anatomical landmarks with echocardiographic and/or fluoroscopic guidance are used to insert the catheter using a Seldinger technique. This can be done in an awake patient with supplemental local anaesthetic and is the treatment of choice for an iatrogenic tamponade caused in the interventional suite [38]. The subcostal approach is safest for a blind procedure in the emergency setting where TTE may not be available. The apical and parasternal approaches may also be used. Pericardiocentesis is diagnostic and therapeutic as drained fluid can be sent for testing. It is the preferred method of drainage in hypotensive patients.

Percutaneous balloon pericardiotomy is performed in a similar manner to TTE-guided pericardiocentesis and is effective in patients with malignant effusions. A balloon is used to generate a pericardial window to prevent recurrence of the tamponade.

Surgical procedures include a pericardial window performed via a substernal approach. Anterolateral thoracotomy and video-assisted thoracoscopic approaches may also be used. Surgical drainage allows for the formation of a pleuropericardial window which allows ongoing drainage of the effusion and decreases the risk of recurrent tamponade. Surgical drainage is preferred for haemopericardium, purulent effusions and recurrent disease. The sub-xiphoid approach consists of a small sub-xiphoid incision made to relieve pressure and directly visualise the parietal pericardium. The advantages of this approach include its effectiveness and simplicity and that it can be performed under local anaesthesia if needed for the patient nearing cardiovascular collapse.

4.1.3 Complications of drainage procedures

Needle pericardiocentesis under ultrasound guidance is considered a life-saving procedure with morbidity rates of 1–3% and a mortality rate of <1% [21, 41, 42, 50].

Puncture and/or rupture of myocardium or coronary vessels; arrhythmias; myocardial infarction; subsequent infection or damage to surrounding structures such as the stomach, liver or lung; and re-accumulation are some of the rare complications.

In the case of a loculated effusion, the pericardiocentesis may not be effective in relieving the chamber compression, and more definitive surgery may be needed.

Paradoxical haemodynamic deterioration following relief of pericardial tamponade is sometimes encountered because of vasovagal effects with decreases in blood pressure and heart rate.

Pericardial decompression syndrome [21, 50] is defined as an unexpected decline in haemodynamic parameters associated with pulmonary oedema and global LV dysfunction. It usually occurs following surgical drainage of large, chronic effusions, but the incidence is rare <5%, and in most patients, there is no discernible reason for the ventricular dysfunction observed. The cause is unknown but may be related to increased interventricular interdependence. The sudden increase in preload and ventricular filling causes an abrupt increase in systolic wall stress, myocardial stunning and volume overload with acute left ventricular failure. Sudden increases in left ventricular end-diastolic pressures are transmitted to the pulmonary circulation with increases in pulmonary pressures and extravasation of fluid into the alveoli leading to pulmonary oedema.

4.1.4 Anaesthetic techniques

All patients require adequate peripheral access and standard ASA monitoring prior to any anaesthetic agent being administered [12, 21, 22, 32, 49, 51–54]. It may also be necessary to institute invasive monitoring via arterial and central venous lines when appropriate, ensuring that insertion of the lines does not delay definitive treatment.

The anaesthetic technique chosen will depend on the clinical condition and haemodynamic stability of the patient, any concomitant co-morbidities, the aetiology of the effusion and the procedure being performed. There are some advantages to performing general anaesthesia over local anaesthesia and sedation. Patient comfort is improved, surgical and operating conditions are optimised and TOE may be employed to guide surgery and ensure adequate evacuation of the effusion [21].

Regardless of the technique chosen, the following haemodynamic goals should be adhered to increase cardiac output, maintain heart rate, maintain sinus rhythm, maintain systemic vascular resistance and left ventricular afterload as tamponade is a fixed output state and ensure an appropriate ventilatory strategy to decrease right atrial and pulmonary pressures. This will augment right atrial filling and decrease right ventricular afterload to promote forward flow through the lungs and maintain left-sided filling pressures from the pulmonary veins.

Local anaesthetic infiltration with supplemental sedation using ketamine, midazolam or fentanyl may be sufficient for pericardiocentesis and sub-xiphoid windows in the less stable patients who are co-operative. Midazolam is a potent, short-acting benzodiazepine that may be used to facilitate drainage procedures under local anaesthesia. Doses of 0.01–0.03 mg/kg may be given slowly and titrated to effect. Respiratory depressant effects are exaggerated with concomitant administration of opioids and other central nervous system depressant drugs.

If general anaesthetic is required, haemodynamic goals remain the same as above. Supplemental administration of fluid and/or blood products with vasopressor or inotropic infusions may be required to support cardiac output.

4.1.4.1 Intraoperatively

Induction of anaesthesia may be associated with severe hypotension and subsequent cardiovascular collapse. The suppression of sympathetic drive from induction agents such as propofol or thiopentone causes vasodilation and bradycardia. Coupled with the deleterious effects of mechanical ventilation as described above, induction of anaesthesia may cause cardiovascular collapse in patients at risk.

The avoidance of respiratory depressant drugs and positive pressure ventilation should be the technique of choice if possible. Spontaneous respiration with a volatile agent such as sevoflurane is ideal if tolerated by the patient. Conditions which may preclude inhalational induction include significant aspiration risk, morbid obesity, severe orthopnoea or an unco-operative patient [12].

Sevoflurane is a fluorinated methyl isopropyl ether anaesthetic agent that is non-pungent, causes minimal airway irritation and is well tolerated by awake, spontaneously breathing patients. It causes a dose-dependent decrease in mean arterial pressure by causing vasodilation and reducing systemic vascular resistance. At concentrations of more than 1.5 minimum alveolar concentration (MAC), increases in heart rate may occur. Nominal changes in cardiac output and stroke volume occur with careful titration. Infusions of vasopressor agents may be required to maintain blood pressures while acquiring adequate depth of anaesthesia with a volatile agent. Adequate depth of anaesthesia should be confirmed before any attempts at manipulation of the airway.

IV induction can be used for more stable patients with no evidence of tamponade. Surgical preparation and draping to facilitate emergency drainage is advisable if IV induction is to be used. IV induction agents need to be carefully selected. Ketamine and etomidate are recommended agents of choice as they will have the least vasodilatory effects.

Ketamine is a phencyclidine derivative that induces a dissociative anaesthetic state. The cardiovascular effects mimic those of sympathetic nervous system stimulation. Systemic blood pressure, heart rate and cardiac output are all increased after intravenous induction doses of 1–2 mg/kg which satisfy the haemodynamic goals required in patients with tamponade pathophysiology. Although there is a theoretical concern about increases in right ventricular afterload with ketamine, it has been used safely in patients for both adjunctive sedation and general anaesthesia. Critically ill patients may respond with unexpected decreases in blood pressure and cardiac output, reflecting a depletion of catecholamine stores and the unmasking of ketamine's direct myocardial depressant effects. Caution must therefore be exercised with these patients. In this instance, it may be more appropriate to use local anaesthesia with supplemental sedation doses of ketamine instead.

Etomidate is a unique carboxylated imidazole-containing compound that exerts its anaesthetic effect by binding to the $GABA_A$ receptor and enhancing GABA binding. Myocardial depressant effects are minimal and contractility is preserved. Nominal changes in heart rate, stroke volume and cardiac output are noted after induction doses of 0.3 mg/kg. This superior cardiovascular stability profile makes etomidate the recommended IV induction agent for patients with little or no cardiovascular reserve.

Propofol is a substituted isopropyl phenol which causes rapid onset of anaesthesia at induction doses of 1.5–2.5 mg/kg when administered intravenously. Its mechanism of action is to modulate GABA receptors causing hyperpolarisation and inhibition of the postsynaptic cell membrane. Propofol causes decreases in systemic vascular resistance, negative inotropy and bradycardia. Vasodilation is mediated by the activation of protein kinase C, increased concentrations of nitric oxide and calcium channel-blocking effects at a cellular level. This effect is present on both sides of the vascular system with arterial- and veno-dilation causing decreases in preload and afterload. Propofol has a depressant effect on the heart rate by decreasing the baroreceptor response to a drop in blood pressure [51]. These effects are exaggerated in patients with tamponade, and the use of propofol at induction doses is not recommended.

Potent opioid agonists, such as fentanyl, are recommended for use in varying doses for both sedation and anaesthesia in patients with cardiac tamponade coming for drainage procedures. They exhibit superior cardiac stability when compared with morphine and are useful adjuncts to provide analgesia and reduce the dose of narcotics required.

Inotropic and vasopressor support should be anticipated, immediately available and used as needed to maintain haemodynamic goals at induction of anaesthesia. The positive inotropic effects of catecholamine enhancing drugs may be limited in patients with tamponade [32]. This may be because patients are already operating at maximum sympathetic stimulation as a compensatory mechanism for the low cardiac output state. The choice of inotropic agent will depend on the patient's clinical condition. Those agents with inodilator properties may improve coronary perfusion initially, but no increase in other organ perfusion has been shown. Caution should be exercised and drugs titrated in at low doses with continuous assessment of haemodynamic response. Vasopressor agents are useful to maintain afterload but should be avoided in patients with normal blood pressure as their use may cause further decreases in cardiac output.

4.1.5 Airway management

Securing a definitive airway early and in the safest way possible is recommended. Endotracheal intubation allows for adequate control of ventilation and oxygenation. Mechanical ventilation may increase right ventricular afterload and decrease forward flow through the right ventricular outflow tract. This will in turn increase right ventricular end-diastolic pressures, worsen interventricular septal shift, further compromise left ventricular filling and negatively impact cardiac output. With an appropriate ventilatory strategy, however, the effect of mechanical ventilation can be minimised. The lowest possible inspiratory pressures and PEEP to maintain minute volume and oxygenation should be used [21].

The choice of endotracheal tube will depend on the procedure. For example, one-lung ventilation may be needed to facilitate surgery in thoracotomy and video-assisted thoracoscopic surgery (VATS). The time taken to insert a double-lumen tube and check its position may be detrimental in an unstable patient. Under these circumstances, placing a single-lumen tube with a bronchial blocker may be more appropriate.

If the patient is very unstable, the safest option may be to perform a sub-xiphoid window initially under local anaesthetic to relieve the tamponade. General anaesthesia may then be more safely induced.

4.1.6 Maintenance of anaesthesia

General anaesthesia care including intraoperative acid–base management, correction of electrolyte abnormalities, temperature and glucose control is required as for all high-risk patients coming for a procedure. These patients may present in a decompensated state which negates pre-operative optimisation of their condition. In the case of any emergency surgery, ongoing resuscitation is required even after the patient has been safely anaesthetised.

IV opioids, propofol, ketamine and volatile agents can all be used if they are tolerated and the haemodynamics remain stable. Careful titration of agents rather than specified doses should be employed. Muscle relaxants should only be used once the patient can tolerate positive pressure ventilation. The choice of neuromuscular-blocking agent will depend on the onset and duration of action required. The newer agents from both the aminosteroid and benzylisoquinoline groups of intermediate-acting neuromuscular-blocking agents are appropriate as they do not exhibit significant cardiovascular effects.

Continuous infusions of inotropes and pressors may be needed and must be continued on a case-by-case basis.

Because of surgical handling of the heart, intraoperative arrhythmias are common and should be anticipated. A defibrillator and antiarrhythmic drugs should be immediately available and standard Advanced Cardiac Life Support (ACLS) algorithms employed to manage peri-operative arrhythmias.

Transfusion triggers and the need for intraoperative administration of blood and clotting factors should be discussed and decided by the multidisciplinary team before induction. Ongoing fluid and blood product resuscitation may be required. Adequate haemoglobin levels to ensure optimal oxygen-carrying capacity is needed and should be individualised per case. Peri-operative monitoring of the patient's coagulation status with thromboelastography (TEG) is advised in order to guide targeted administration of plasma products and pharmacological agents that may be required.

Because intrinsic myocardial function is generally preserved in pericardial effusion and tamponade, once the tamponade is relieved, there is usually a dramatic improvement in haemodynamics. At this point, vasopressor and inotropic infusions should be reviewed and weaned if appropriate. The use of vasodilator therapy is controversial and only indicated if there is associated systemic hypertension and elevated systemic vascular resistance [32].

4.1.6.1 Post-operatively

Patients should be transferred to a high-dependency unit for continuation of care. Ongoing monitoring is necessary to assess for recurrence of tamponade, ongoing bleeding and continuation of cardiovascular and ventilatory support.

4.2 Pericardiectomy for constrictive pericarditis

Pericardiectomy is the only definitive treatment for established constriction, and most studies suggest that resection should be as complete as technically feasible [49, 54–57]. A retrospective review by Nozohoor et al. showed that radical pericardiectomy was associated with improved functional status and 10-year survival rates of 94% compared to 55% with subtotal pericardiectomy [55]. Bozbuga et al. also showed that performing early radical resection in combination with appropriate chemotherapeutic agents translated into the best outcomes in patients with tuberculous disease [56].

4.2.1 Types of pericardiectomy

Pericardial stripping is carried out via sternotomy or lateral thoracotomy with or without cardiopulmonary bypass support [49]. Total resection is extremely difficult to perform via a thoracotomy, and median sternotomy is the preferred approach to provide definitive resection and optimise benefit [49, 55].

Partial pericardiectomy is defined as incomplete decortication of one or both ventricles because of severe myo-pericardial adhesions.

Total pericardiectomy is when wide excision of the pericardium is performed. The anatomical borders consist of the phrenic nerves posteriorly, the great vessels and intra-pericardial portion of the superior vena cava/right atrial junction superiorly and the diaphragm and inferior vena cava/right atrial junction inferiorly.

Radical resection is the removal of the pericardium including the anterolateral and diaphragmatic surfaces of the left and right ventricles with careful dissection posterior to the phrenic nerves to leave the left and right phrenic pedicles intact.

Epicardial involvement may be missed at surgery leading to persistent constrictive physiology post-operatively. Reoperation to remove the diseased epicardium or visceral pericardium may be required [49].

The need for cardiopulmonary bypass (CPB) should be individualised per case. Studies suggest that mortality rates are higher in patients who required CPB, but data may be skewed because its use is usually reserved for patients with a poor pre-operative status. Other indications include any coexisting cardiac conditions that may require intervention, previous cardiac surgery or partial pericardiectomy, a heavily calcified pericardial "cocoon" encasing all four cardiac chambers, post mediastinal irradiation and unintentional surgical damage to cardiac structures intraoperatively [49].

Persistent constrictive physiology and abnormal diastolic filling patterns may be seen in a percentage of patients even after successful surgery. In conjunction with symptomatic improvement, normalisation of pressure-volume loops and echocardiographic findings post pericardiectomy are used as markers of successful resection [49, 58].

4.2.2 Complications associated with pericardiectomy

Pericardiectomy is a very technically challenging operation with significant morbidity and mortality performed in high-risk patients [49, 54–57, 59]. Intraoperative complications may contribute significantly to poor outcomes. Sufficient pre-operative preparation prior to induction of anaesthesia is paramount to ensuring patient safety, and a multidisciplinary team approach should be used.

Massive haemorrhage should be anticipated with contingency plans in place before the administration of any anaesthetic agents. Timeous activation of a massive transfusion protocol is necessary. Cardiopulmonary bypass support should be immediately available with cannulation of femoral vessels under local anaesthesia in select patients with severe or decompensated disease. Appropriate IV access and invasive monitoring should be established, and inotropic or vasopressor infusions drawn up and running at the time of induction of anaesthesia. Damage to underlying epicardium, myocardium and coronary vessels poses the most risk to patients contributing to an overall mortality of about 7–18% [4]. Arrhythmias are common and prompt management as per the latest ACLS guidelines.

Low cardiac output syndrome, defined as a cardiac index of <2.2 l/min/m, will result in a subset of patients with chronic constrictive pericarditis [49, 60]. This is a form of acute cardiac failure, and there are a number of suggested mechanisms. The underlying myocardium may be affected by prolonged constriction causing myocardial disuse atrophy; residual constriction from partial or incomplete removal of the epicardial layer results in persistent constriction; the disease process itself may affect the myocardium; prolonged abnormal diastolic filling leads to architectural changes with remodelling of the ventricles; worsening of tricuspid regurgitation with progressive right ventricular dysfunction causes volume overload and right ventricular failure; and elongation of the papillary muscles leads to significant mitral regurgitation and left ventricular failure post relief of the constriction.

The incidence of low cardiac output syndrome post pericardiectomy is 28% with an associated mortality rate of up to 70% [60, 61]. Patients demonstrating prolonged symptomatic disease are at greatest risk [60]. This complication should be anticipated peri-operatively and managed with the appropriate haemodynamic and ventilatory support. Some studies suggest that levosimendan may be a pharmacological agent of choice [60].

4.2.3 Anaesthetic management

Intraoperative haemodynamic goals are to maintain heart rate, maintain systemic vascular resistance, optimise venous return and support myocardial contractility [12, 21, 22, 32, 49, 51–54, 60]. General anaesthesia care including intraoperative acid–base management, correction of electrolyte abnormalities, temperature and glucose control is required and will apply to these patients as mentioned above for pericardial tamponade.

Because CP is a fixed output state, patients have an increased reliance on heart rate and systemic vascular resistance to maintain systolic blood pressures and organ perfusion. Optimisation of preload and venous return preinduction are important to compensate for the decreased filling of the cardiac chambers. The consequences of possible fluid overload must always be considered, and these patients require dynamic assessment of fluid status as they too operate at the lower end of the Frank-Starling curve. This places them at increased risk for volume overload and low cardiac output syndrome, especially after relief of the constriction.

A balanced anaesthetic technique ensuring haemodynamic goals is necessary to avoid sudden decompensation at induction of anaesthesia [54, 60]. Ketamine is often recommended as the anaesthetic induction agent of choice because of its sympathomimetic effects on the cardiovascular system. Midazolam, etomidate and potent opioids such as fentanyl have also been safely used for induction of anaesthesia. Securing a definitive airway is recommended, and the use of muscle relaxants can be used early on, bearing in mind the possible deleterious effects of mechanical ventilation. The institution of positive pressure ventilation may compromise right heart chamber filling, and appropriate settings are needed to optimise ventilation, oxygenation and haemodynamics.

It is highly recommended that inotropic and/or vasopressor infusions are drawn up and running at the time of induction. These should be continued and titrated throughout surgery and continued into the post-operative period in anticipation for a persistent low cardiac output state, especially in at-risk patients.

Anticipation for massive blood loss, both acute and ongoing, is of vital importance as mentioned above. Monitoring with heightened intraoperative vigilance, regular blood gas and TEG analysis will guide transfusion of blood, clotting factors and pharmacological agents that may be required.

Damage to cardiac structures may lead to massive sudden haemorrhage, myocardial ischaemia or significant arrhythmias. Appropriate management must be instituted immediately and may include the need for cardiopulmonary bypass if conventional surgical and medical management fail.

The need for elective cardiopulmonary bypass support will depend on the pre-operative condition of the patient, the aetiology of the CP and the underlying myocardial function. The decision for the adjunctive use of bypass should be discussed and decided upon during the multidisciplinary team discussion prior to surgery. If deemed necessary, the femoral vessels should be prepped and cannulated under local anaesthesia prior to induction of anaesthesia.

Post-operatively, patients should be transferred to a high-dependency unit for continuation of care. Ongoing monitoring for persistent bleeding and low cardiac output syndrome is necessary as well as ongoing haemodynamic and ventilatory support.

4.2.4 Predictors of outcome following pericardiectomy

Early post-operative mortality rates are in the region of 18% [46, 49, 56, 57, 59]. Peri-operative mortality is highly dependent on the patient's pre-operative NYHA status [56].

Predictors of poor long-term outcome include the aetiology of the disease, previous radiation, renal dysfunction, hyponatraemia, old age, low pre-operative left ventricular ejection fraction, right ventricular dilatation, elevated pulmonary pressures and the severity of tricuspid regurgitation [46, 49, 57, 59].

Because of the high peri-operative morbidity and mortality, patients with mild or very advanced disease, renal failure or post-radiation constrictive pericarditis should be evaluated very carefully pre-operatively as the risk of pericardiectomy may outweigh the benefits.

5. Conclusion

Patients with pericardial disease can be challenging for the attending anaesthesiologist. An in-depth understanding of the pathophysiology of each disease state is necessary to provide optimal care. Careful pre-operative evaluation of the clinical history, examination and diagnostic investigations will allow adequate evaluation of risk and alert the anaesthesiologist to the necessary steps to be taken to manage these high-risk patients in the safest way possible.

An appreciation of how the chosen anaesthetic technique may influence the patient's haemodynamic state is necessary to avoid unwanted anaesthetic complications. This includes a thorough understanding of the effect of pharmacological agents as well as how mechanical ventilation may influence haemodynamics. The potential risk and complications of the surgical procedure should be examined and discussed with the multidisciplinary team pre-operatively in order to ensure adequate preparation for any potentially catastrophic events. These patients are best cared for by experienced peri-operative teams who have this appreciation.

Author details

Michelle Correia
Department of Anaesthesiology and Pain Medicine, Nelson Mandela Children's Hospital, University of the Witwatersrand, Johannesburg, Gauteng, South Africa

*Address all correspondence to: michelle.correia@nmch.org.za

IntechOpen

© 2019 The Author(s). Licensee IntechOpen. This chapter is distributed under the terms of the Creative Commons Attribution License (http://creativecommons.org/licenses/by/3.0), which permits unrestricted use, distribution, and reproduction in any medium, provided the original work is properly cited.

References

[1] Rodriguez ER, Tan CD. Structure and anatomy of the human pericardium. Progress in Cardiovascular Diseases. 2017;**59**(4):327-340

[2] Peebles CR, Shambrook JS, Harden SP. Pericardial disease—Anatomy and function. The British Journal of Radiology. 2011;**84**(special_issue_3):S324-S337

[3] Little WC, Freeman GL. Pericardial disease. Circulation. 2006;**113**(12):1622-1632

[4] Goldstein JA. Cardiac tamponade, constrictive pericarditis, and restrictive cardiomyopathy. Current Problems in Cardiology. 2004;**29**(9):503-567

[5] Collins D. Aetiology and management of acute cardiac tamponade. Critical Care and Resuscitation. 2004;**6**(1):54

[6] Adler Y, Charron P, Imazio M, Badano L, Barón Esquivias G, Bogaert J, et al. 2015 ESC Guidelines for the diagnosis and management of pericardial diseases: The Task Force for the Diagnosis and Management of Pericardial Diseases of the European Society of Cardiology (ESC) Endorsed by: The European Association for Cardio-Thoracic Surgery (EACTS). European Heart Journal. 2015;**36**(42):2921-2964

[7] Hoit BD. Pericardial disease and pericardial tamponade. Critical Care Medicine. 2007;**35**(8):S355-S364

[8] Anesthetic Considerations for Patients with Pericardial Disease. Available from: https://aneskey.com/anesthetic-considerations- for-patients-with-pericardial-disease/

[9] Ristic A, Simeunovic D. Preoperative and perioperative management of patients with pericardial diseases. Acta Chirurgica Iugoslavica. 2011;**LVIII**:45-53

[10] Anesthetic Pericarditis, Pericardial Tamponade, and Myocarditis. Available from: https://aneskey.com/pericarditis-pericardial- tamponade-and-myocarditis/

[11] Lange RA, Hillis LD. Acute pericarditis. The New England Journal of Medicine. 2004;**351**(21):2195-2202

[12] Grocott HP, Gulati H, Srinathan S, Mackensen GB. Anesthesia and the patient with pericardial disease. Canadian Journal of Anesthesia/Journal canadien d'anesthésie. 2011;**58**(10):952

[13] Imazio M, Hoit BD. Post-cardiac injury syndromes. An emerging cause of pericardial diseases. International Journal of Cardiology. 2013;**168**(2):648-652

[14] Tamarappoo BK, Klein AL. Post-pericardiotomy syndrome. Current Cardiology Reports. 2016;**18**(11):116

[15] Imazio M, Bobbio M, Cecchi E, Demarie D, Pomari F, Moratti M, et al. Colchicine as first-choice therapy for recurrent pericarditis: Results of the CORE (COlchicine for REcurrent pericarditis) trial. Archives of Internal Medicine. 2005;**165**(17):1987-1991

[16] Imazio M, Brucato A, Cumetti D, Brambilla G, Demichelis B, Ferro S, et al. Corticosteroids for recurrent pericarditis: High versus low doses: A nonrandomized observation. Circulation. 2008;**118**(6):667-671

[17] Syed FF, Mayosi BM. A modern approach to tuberculous pericarditis. Progress in Cardiovascular Diseases. 2007;**50**(3):218-236

[18] Rehman KA, Betancor J, Xu B, Kumar A, Rivas CG, Sato K, et al. Uremic pericarditis, pericardial effusion, and constrictive pericarditis

in end-stage renal disease: Insights and pathophysiology. Clinical Cardiology. 2017;**40**(10):839-846

[19] Alpert MA, Ravenscraft MD. Pericardial involvement in end-stage renal disease. The American Journal of the Medical Sciences. 2003;**325**(4):228-236

[20] Leehey DJ, Daugirdas JT, Popli S, Gandhi VC, Pifarre R, Ing TS. Predicting need for surgical drainage of pericardial effusion in patients with end-stage renal disease. The International Journal of Artificial Organs. 1989;**12**(10):618-625

[21] O'Connor CJ, Tuman KJ. The intraoperative management of patients with pericardial tamponade. Anesthesiology Clinics. 2010;**28** (1, 1):87-96

[22] Odor P, Bailey A. Cardiac tamponade. Anaesthesia tutorial of the week 283. ATOTW 283—Cardiac Tamponade. 2013. Available from: https://www.wfsahq.org/components/com_virtual_library/media/1b3d4f771bc9361a73764d03a184cf76-283-Cardiac-Tamponade-RFS.pdf

[23] Bodson L, Bouferrache K, Vieillard-Baron A. Cardiac tamponade. Current Opinion in Critical Care. 2011;**17**(5):416-424

[24] Spodick DH. Acute cardiac tamponade. The New England Journal of Medicine. 2003;**349**(7):684-690

[25] Grecu L. Cardiac tamponade. International Anesthesiology Clinics. 2012;**50**(2):59-77

[26] Kronzon I, Cohen ML, Winer HE. Diastolic atrial compression: A sensitive echocardiographic sign of cardiac tamponade. Journal of the American College of Cardiology. 1983;**2**(4):770-775

[27] Reydel B, Spodick DH. Frequency and significance of chamber collapses during cardiac tamponade. American Heart Journal. 1990;**119**(5):1160-1163

[28] Leeman DE, Levine MJ, Come PC. Doppler echocardiography in cardiac tamponade: Exaggerated respiratory variation in transvalvular blood flow velocity integrals. Journal of the American College of Cardiology. 1988;**11**(3):572-578

[29] Magder S, Erice F, Lagonidis D. Determinants of the Y descent and its usefulness as a predictor of ventricular filling. Journal of Intensive Care Medicine. 2000;**15**(5):262-269

[30] Pepi M, Muratori M. Echocardiography in the diagnosis and management of pericardial disease. Journal of Cardiovascular Medicine. 2006;7(7):533-544

[31] Verhaert D, Gabriel RS, Johnston D, Lytle BW, Desai MY, Klein AL. The role of multimodality imaging in the management of pericardial disease. Circulation. Cardiovascular Imaging. 2010;**3**(3):333-343

[32] Carmona P, Mateo E, Casanovas I, Peña JJ, Llagunes J, Aguar F, et al. Management of cardiac tamponade after cardiac surgery. Journal of Cardiothoracic and Vascular Anesthesia. 2012;**26**(2):302-311

[33] Khan NK, Järvelä KM, Loisa EL, Sutinen JA, Laurikka JO, Khan JA. Incidence, presentation and risk factors of late postoperative pericardial effusions requiring invasive treatment after cardiac surgery. Interactive Cardiovascular and Thoracic Surgery. 2017;**24**:835-840

[34] Ashikhmina EA, Schaff HV, Sinak LJ, Li Z, Dearani JA, Suri RM, et al. Pericardial effusion after cardiac surgery: Risk factors, patient profiles, and contemporary management. The Annals of thoracic surgery. 2010;**89**(1):112-118

[35] Pompilio G, Filippini S, Agrifoglio M, Merati E, Lauri G, Salis S, et al. Determinants of pericardial drainage for cardiac tamponade following cardiac surgery. European Journal of Cardio-Thoracic Surgery. 2011;**39**(5):e107-e113

[36] Pepi M, Muratori M, Barbier P, Doria E, Arena V, Berti M, et al. Pericardial effusion after cardiac surgery: Incidence, site, size, and haemodynamic consequences. Heart. 1994;**72**(4):327-331

[37] Kuvin JT, Harati NA, Pandian NG, Bojar RM, Khabbaz KR. Postoperative cardiac tamponade in the modern surgical era. The Annals of thoracic surgery. 2002;**74**(4):1148-1153

[38] Floerchinger B, Camboni D, Schopka S, Kolat P, Hilker M, Schmid C. Delayed cardiac tamponade after open heart surgery-is supplemental CT imaging reasonable? Journal of Cardiothoracic Surgery. 2013;**8**(1):158

[39] Holmes DR Jr, Nishimura R, Fountain R, Turi ZG. Iatrogenic pericardial effusion and tamponade in the percutaneous intracardiac intervention era. JACC. Cardiovascular Interventions. 2009;**2**(8):705-717

[40] Fejka M, Dixon SR, Safian RD, O'Neill WW, Grines CL, Finta B, et al. Diagnosis, management, and clinical outcome of cardiac tamponade complicating percutaneous coronary intervention. The American Journal of Cardiology. 2002;**90**(11):1183-1186

[41] Bauer T, Boeder N, Nef HM, Möllmann H, Hochadel M, Marco J, et al. Fate of patients with coronary perforation complicating percutaneous coronary intervention (from the Euro Heart Survey Percutaneous Coronary Intervention Registry). The American Journal of Cardiology. 2015;**116**(9):1363-1367

[42] Kumar R, Sinha A, Lin MJ, Uchino R, Butryn T, O'Mara MS, et al. Complications of pericardiocentesis: A clinical synopsis. International Journal of Critical Illness and Injury Science. 2015;**5**(3):206

[43] Bertog SC, Thambidorai SK, Parakh K, Schoenhagen P, Ozduran V, Houghtaling PL, et al. Constrictive pericarditis: Etiology and cause-specific survival after pericardiectomy. Journal of the American College of Cardiology. 2004;**43**(8):1445-1452

[44] Skubas NJ, Beardslee M, Barzilai B, Pasque M, Kattapuram M, Lappas DG. Constrictive pericarditis: Intraoperative hemodynamic and echocardiographic evaluation of cardiac filling dynamics. Anesthesia and Analgesia. 2001;**92**(6):1424-1426

[45] Santamore WP, Bartlett R, Van Buren SJ, Dowd MK, Kutcher MA. Ventricular coupling in constrictive pericarditis. Circulation. 1986;**74**(3):597-602

[46] Schwefer M, Aschenbach R, Heidemann J, Mey C, Lapp H. Constrictive pericarditis, still a diagnostic challenge: Comprehensive review of clinical management. European Journal of Cardio-Thoracic Surgery. 2009;**36**(3):502-510

[47] Hoit BD, LeWinter MM, Aldea GS, Verrier E, Downey BC. Constrictive pericarditis. In: LeWinter MM, Aldea GS, Verrier E, section editors. Up to date. 2011. Available from: https://www.uptodate.com/contents/constrictive-pericarditis

[48] Talreja DR, Edwards WD, Danielson GK, et al. Constrictive pericarditis in 26 patients with histologically normal pericardial thickness. Circulation. 2003;**108**:1852-1857

[49] Chowdhury UK, Sankhyan LK. Pericardiectomy for chronic constrictive pericarditis: Where are we after 100 years. World Journal of Surgery and Surgical Research. 2018;**1**:1027

[50] Imazio M. Pericardial decompression syndrome: A rare but potentially fatal complication of pericardial drainage to be recognized and prevented. European Heart Journal of Acute Cardiovascular Care. 2015;**4**(2):121-123

[51] Stoelting RK, Hillier SC. Pharmacology and Physiology in Anesthetic Practice. 2nd ed. Wolters Kluwer, Lippincott Williams & Wilkins; 2006

[52] Aye T, Milne B. Ketamine anesthesia for pericardial window in a patient with pericardial tamponade and severe COPD. Canadian Journal of Anesthesia. 2002;**49**(3):283

[53] Bilotta F, Fiorani L, La Rosa I, Spinelli F, Rosa G. Cardiovascular effects of intravenous propofol administered at two infusion rates: A transthoracic echocardiographic study. Anaesthesia. 2001;**56**(3):266-271

[54] Jasper AO, Anyanhun GA, Okugbo SU, Adudu P. Pericardiectomy in post-traumatic suppurative constrictive pericarditis: Case report. Cases Journal. 2009;**2**(1):9292

[55] Nozohoor S, Johansson M, Koul B, Cunha-Goncalves D. Radical pericardiectomy for chronic constrictive pericarditis. Journal of Cardiac Surgery. Jun 2018;**33**(6):301-307

[56] Bozbuga N, Erentug V, Eren E, Erdogan HB, Kirali K, Antal A, et al. Pericardiectomy for chronic constrictive tuberculous pericarditis: Risks and predictors of survival. Texas Heart Institute Journal. 2003;**30**(3):180

[57] Biçer M, Özdemir B, Kan İ, Yüksel A, Tok M, Şenkaya I. Long-term outcomes of pericardiectomy for constrictive pericarditis. Journal of Cardiothoracic Surgery. 2015;**10**(1):177

[58] Patil DV, Sabnis GR, Phadke MS, Lanjewar CP, Mishra P, Kulkarni DV, et al. Echocardiographic parameters in clinical responders to surgical pericardiectomy—A single center experience with chronic constrictive pericarditis. Indian Heart Journal. 2016;**68**(3):316-324

[59] Busch C, Penov K, Amorim PA, Garbade J, Davierwala P, Schuler GC, et al. Risk factors for mortality after pericardiectomy for chronic constrictive pericarditis in a large single-centre cohort. European Journal of Cardio-Thoracic Surgery. 2015;**48**(6):e110-e116

[60] Nath MP, Barman M, Bhattacharrya RK. Severe low cardiac output following pericardiectomy-bird in cage phenomenon. Journal of Vascular Medicine & Surgery. 2014;**14**:2014

[61] McCaughan BC, Schaff HV, Piehler JM, Danielson GK, Orszulak TA, Puga FJ, et al. Early and late results of pericardiectomy for constrictive pericarditis. The Journal of Thoracic and Cardiovascular Surgery. 1985;**89**(3):340-350

Section 2

Cardiomyopathies

Chapter 7

Inflammation and Diabetic Cardiomyopathy

Manal M.A. Smail, Chris F. Howarth, Jaipaul Singh and Abla Mohamed Ismail

Abstract

Diabetes mellitus (DM) is a metabolic syndrome that manifests a low grade of systemic inflammation that contributes to the development of cardiovascular diseases (CVDs). DM is a predominant risk factor for CVDs inducing structural changes in the heart, infiltration of fibrosis, apoptosis, and cardiac remodeling, all leading to myocardial infarction (MI), heart failure (HF), and sudden cardiac death. Furthermore, more than 80% of diabetic patients usually die from heart diseases or diabetic cardiomyopathy (DCM). Currently, HF is one of the main causes of mortality in the world despite advances in drug treatments. According to literature, a strong association exists between chronic inflammation and the development of DCM. In order to have a better appreciation of the effect of diabetes and inflammation on the cardiovascular system (CVS), it is of paramount importance to have a better understanding of diabetes, the physiology of the CVS, and the pathophysiology of DM. Thus, the present review highlights the role of chronic inflammation in the complex interplay between the development of DM and DCM. Our understanding of the process is critical in the discovery of new targeted therapies for DCM and other forms of HF.

Keywords: heart, cardiomyopathy, hyperglycaemia, hypertension, inflammation

1. Introduction

Cardiovascular diseases (CVDs) remain the leading cause of death in the world [1, 2]. By the year 2020, it is estimated that nearly 40% of all deaths worldwide will be due to CVDs, more than twice the percentage of deaths from cancer [3]. In line with the 2017 Update: A Report From the American Heart Association, CVDs account for one out of every three deaths or approximately 800,000 deaths in the United States, and coronary heart disease (CHD) accounts for most deaths due to CVDs, followed by stroke (1 of 20 deaths in the United States) and heart failure (HF) [4]. CVDs are considered multifactorial conditions which affect the essential components of the circulatory system of the human body including the heart, blood vessels and blood [5]. CVDs can either be congenital or acquired throughout people's lifespan [6]. The rising incidence of such cardiovascular risk factors as unhealthy life styles (especially eating and physical inactivity), obesity, diabetes and hypertension can underlie an increase in CVDs especially coronary artery disease (CAD). The burden of chronic diseases, including CVDs, obesity, diabetes and cancers, is rapidly increasing worldwide. These non-communicable diseases have become a major health concern and burden to mankind, not just in developed countries but also in developing countries [7]. Chronic inflammation and oxidative stress are associated with the development of various CVDs including hypertension, arrhythmias, CAD and HF. Globally, CVDs remain a leading cause of death despite the development of new drugs and novel treatments [2]. Recent data showed that the prevalence of macro-vascular complications including coronary artery disease (CAD), peripheral artery disease (PAD) and stroke is two to four times more common in people with diabetes than healthy subjects [8]. According to the Framingham Study, the frequency of CAD is twice as common in diabetic patients of both sexes [1]. Existing data highlight the complex nature of the cardiovascular system, and different signalling pathways may play various roles depending on the stages of the pathology. In order to have a better appreciation of the effect of CVDs on the increased morbidity and mortality rate, it is helpful to have a brief understanding of the physiology and pathophysiology of the cardiovascular system.

2. Cardiovascular system physiology and pathophysiology

The cardiovascular system (CVS) is composed of the blood, heart and blood vessels. The heart is a relentless muscular organ, which never stops pumping blood during life. It beats approximately 100,000 times per day, and each beat requires a vast amount of energy. The weight of the human heart is around 250–300 g for adult and a size similar to a closed fist. The heart rests on the diaphragm, near the midline of the thoracic cavity, and is surrounded by a fibrous sac called the pericardium [9]. The heart is divided into left and right sides by a septal wall. Each side of the heart is made up of two chambers, the atria and ventricles which are separated by atrioventricular valves [9]. The left side of the heart delivers oxygen-rich blood to the body passing through the aortic valve to the aorta (systemic circulation), while the right side pumps blood to the lungs passing though the pulmonary valve and the pulmonary artery for oxygen replenishment in the lungs (pulmonary circulation). The four valves of the heart ensure unidirectional flow of blood through the heart. The valves are opened and closed due to pressure differences between the heart chambers. The right atrium receives deoxygenated blood from the body through the superior and inferior vena cavae, while the left atrium receives oxygenated blood from the lungs through pulmonary veins. Coronary arteries supply the myocardium with oxygen-rich blood (the left anterior descending coronary artery, the left circumflex artery and the right coronary artery). The apex of the heart is the pointed end, and the area opposite the apex is called the base of the heart [10]. HF develops when the volume of blood pumped from the heart is inadequate to meet the metabolic demands or needs of the body [11]. The traditional hemodynamic hypothesis is that diseases, which normally increase the hemodynamic burden of the heart, ultimately lead to HF by inducing defects in the contractility of cardiac myocytes. The hypothesis of depressed cardiac myocyte contractility in HF is in support of several other related studies [12, 13], but not all [14]. Previous investigations suggested that cardiac myocytes in the failing human heart undergo many alterations which result in a significant loss of contractile function. These alterations involved a reduction in α-myosin heavy chain gene expression along with a rise in β-myosin heavy chain gene expression, significant loss of myofilaments in myocytes and changes in cytoskeletal proteins [15].

There is general agreement about the contractile properties of the myocardium, which can be similar in both normal and in failing heart muscle under basal conditions. However, the rate-related contractile reserve is absent or significantly reduced in failing human myocardium [16]. Many studies reported that during the end-stage of HF, basal contractility is well preserved, but the ability to increase contractility with heart rate or sympathetic stimulation is severely depressed [17]. Thus, the fundamental changes in muscle performance and regulation can be explained by the poor pumping function, reduced exercise capacity and tachycardia intolerance of the human failing heart [14]. HF can no longer be considered a simple contractile disorder or a disease of the heart alone [18]. Clinical manifestations are, in fact, the result of changes to the cellular, sub-cellular and molecular components of the heart and to mediators that drive homeostatic control mechanisms. Cardiac remodelling (CR) is now generally accepted as a determinant of the clinical course of HF. CR is defined as genome expression, resulting in molecular, cellular and interstitial changes, and manifested clinically as changes in size, shape and function of the heart. CR is determined by the general process of adaptation, which allows for both the myocyte and the collagen network to adapt to new working conditions [19].

3. Inflammation

Inflammation is one of the body's defence mechanisms, and there are commonly two types of inflammation, namely, acute and chronic inflammation. Acute inflammation starts rapidly and becomes more severe in a short time, and the symptoms may last for a few days. On the other hand, chronic inflammation which is a long-term inflammation in nature can last for prolonged periods of several months to years. Generally, the extent and effects of chronic inflammation vary with the cause of the injury and the ability of the body to repair and overcome the damage [4]. This review now describes the relevant data about inflammation induced by several risk factors leading to the onset of CVDs. Basically, an inflammatory response aims to reduce the agent that causes tissue injury and to induce appropriate wound healing and to restore tissue homeostasis [20]. A cascade of inflammatory pathways and mechanistic effects are supposedly well-orchestrated by the immune system in order to eradicate the causative agent. Several immune cells can change their number, morphology and nature depending on the stage and type of inflammation [20], provided that the immune response succeeds in repairing the initial tissue injury. However, in cases where the inflammation fails to resolve, the tissue injury, due to the persistence of the triggering agent(s) or due to unsuccessful repair of the initial tissue injury or dysfunction, a sustained underlying inflammatory process can develop, leading to further tissue dysfunction and detrimental consequences [21]. Several traditional and emerging risk factors are thought to influence the cardiovascular system especially inflammation-related chronic diseases, by their interrelation with underlying molecular and cellular manifestations. In turn, these can result in chronic inflammatory responses leading to the loss of tissue properties and subsequently dysfunction [22]. Apart from dyslipidaemia, other well-established risk factors are involved in the process including hypertension, diabetes and obesity. Inflammation that causes endothelial dysfunction seems to be the key causative underlying mechanistic player, at the molecular and cellular levels, for the onset and development of subsequent inflammation-related chronic disorders such as atherosclerosis and subsequent CVDs and renal disorders [23, 24]. Hypertension, diabetes and obesity have harmful effects of oxidised low-density lipoprotein cholesterol, initiating a chronic inflammatory reaction, the result of which is a vulnerable plaque, prone to rupture and thrombosis. Epidemiological and clinical studies have shown strong and consistent relationships between markers of inflammation and risk of future cardiovascular events [3]. Inflammation is widely considered to be an important contributing factor in atherogenesis and the risk of athero-thrombotic complications. Baseline measurements of some inflammatory markers are well-known to be predictive risk factors for future CVD events in prospective epidemiological studies. Inflammatory markers dominant in the literature are acute phase response (APR)-associated, and they include fibrinogen and C-reactive protein (CRP) [25].

The presence of subclinical inflammation is accompanied by an elevated concentration of high-sensitivity CRP and increased concentrations of other inflammatory markers. Epidemiological studies suggest strong association between high-sensitivity CRP concentrations and CVD risks [37].

4. Risk factors for cardiovascular diseases

There are a number causal risk factors which are associated with CVDs and it is of paramount importance to understand and recognise these risk factors in order to predict and more so, to prevent CVDs. Risk factors may be causal or just a marker of risk(s) in nature and they are often called "innocent bystanders" [26]. The WHO has identified high blood pressure, tobacco use, physical inactivity, unhealthy diet, overweight, obesity, diabetes, high blood glucose and high cholesterol, as the main causal factors of the global burden of CVDs [27]. This review will now focus on how hypertension and diabetes mellitus can lead to heart failure (HF) and diabetes-induced cardiomyopathy (DCM).

5. Hypertension and ischaemic heart disease

Hypertension is a well-recognised risk factor for CVDs [28]. In fact, 14 weeks of hypertension can increase left ventricular weight by 30% and wall thickness by 42%, while the number of myocytes and total length of capillaries remain constant. Hypertrophy of myocytes is associated with reduced mitochondria to myofibril ratio [29]. Thus, physiological and pathological cardiac hypertrophies are caused by different stimuli and functionally distinguishable. A pathological stimulus causing pressure overload like hypertension produces an increase in systolic wall stress which results in in concentric hypertrophy (a heart with a very thick wall but with relatively small cavities) [30]. In the pathological hypertrophied heart, the function may decompensate, resulting in left ventricle dilation and HF. However, in physiological hypertrophy, the function does not decompensate [30]. Accordingly, regular exercise training (ET) can induce beneficial effects in the myocardium. Cardiac action potential duration (CAPD) of the hypertrophied heart is prolonged compared to control [31]. According to literature, mortality rates from coronary artery and cerebrovascular diseases can increase progressively as blood pressure increases [21]. CAD is caused by the accumulation of lipid and inflammatory cells in the arterial walls to form atherosclerotic plaques. Unstable coronary plaques are prone to erosion or rupture, obstructing coronary blood flow and causing an acute myocardial infraction (MI). It is now known that various CVDs can alter the ultrastructure of the heart. Myocardial ischaemia develops when the coronary blood supply to the myocardium is reduced either in terms of absolute flow rate (low-flow or no flow) or relative to increased tissue demand. The main feature of ischaemia is that oxygen supply to the mitochondria is insufficient to support oxidative phosphorylation [32]. After the onset of ischaemia, ultrastructural changes in the myocardium occur rapidly. These changes can be considered as reversible alterations if reperfusion of the tissue can be effected quickly. However, when ischaemia lasts for more than 20–30 min without collateral flow, the result is a transition from a state of reversible ultrastructural alterations to a state of irreversible tissue injury [33]. An early consequence of myocardial ischaemia is depression of myocardial contractility. Also during ischaemia, arrhythmias may occur, ranging in severity from isolated ventricular premature beats, through runs of ventricular tachycardia, to ventricular fibrillation [34]. During ischaemia, there is a reduced availability of oxygen and the metabolic substrates, leading to a deficit of high-energy phosphates. In addition, the Ca^{2+} uptake mechanisms in the sarcoplasmic reticulum (SR) of cardiac myocytes are impaired, leading to intracellular free Ca^{2+} accumulation or elevated diastolic $[Ca^{2+}]_i$ [35].

6. Diabetes induced cardiomyopathy (DCM)

CVDs are closely associated with diabetes-induced hyperglycaemia, resulting in the death in 80% of people with diabetes [1]. Diabetic cardiomyopathy (DCM) is defined as a disorder of the heart muscle caused by diabetes. It results in pathological cardiac remodelling without previous incidence of CAD, hypertension and valvular disease. The exact cellular, subcellular and molecular mechanisms of DCM are complex and remain unclear [2]. Thus, further studies are essential for better understanding of the mechanism(s) of DCM and also in reversing the pathological cardiac remodelling induced by diabetes [3]. The increased frequency of HF in diabetic patients can persist despite correction for age, obesity, hypercholesterolemia and CAD. DCM is characterized by diastolic dysfunction, which can lead to the development of systolic dysfunction [36]. Echocardiography for patients with type 1 diabetes mellitus (T1DM) without known CAD shows diastolic dysfunction with a reduction in early diastolic filling, increase in atrial filling, an extension of iso-volumetric relation and increased numbers of supra-ventricular premature beats. The most common abnormality observed in asymptomatic diabetics is left ventricular (LV) diastolic dysfunction, likely resulting from greater LV myocardial and vascular stiffness [37]. A deep understanding of its development is necessary for the early diagnosis and subsequent treatment of diabetes-related cardiovascular diseases.

There is a rapidly growing literature on DCM investigating the structural, functional and metabolic changes that occur in the diabetic myocardium and how these changes contribute to the development of DCM in humans [38, 39]. The structural changes include left ventricular hypertrophy, interstitial fibrosis, increased cell death and oxidative stress and myocardial lipotoxicity [40, 41]. The functional changes include diastolic dysfunction, systolic dysfunction and impaired contractile reserve. Metabolic changes include altered substrate utilisation and mitochondrial dysfunction [42]. In type 2 diabetes mellitus (T2DM), left ventricular mass is an independent marker of cardiovascular risks that often occur independently of atrial blood pressure. Hence, diabetes is an independent risk factor leading to left ventricular hypertrophy, myocardial stiffness and inflammation [43]. DCM is also characterized by interstitial fibrosis, mostly composed of collagen and perivascular fibrosis [44]. In biopsies from diabetic heart patients, the deposition of collagen around the vessel and between myofibres is significantly raised. Furthermore, lipofuscin (which is a brown pigment composed of lipid-containing residues), cholesterol and myocardial triglyceride is also significantly increased in cardiac tissue biopsies from the left ventricle [45].

During DCM, hyperglycaemia (HG) can lead to both acute reversible cellular metabolism damage and irreversible changes in endogenous macromolecules in the heart [46]. Elevated blood HG can affect many organs in the body including the kidneys, the eyes, the nerves and the heart resulting in long-term damage and failure [47, 48]. The first target of HG-induced damage is the microvasculature. As a result, the small blood vessels will initiate a systematic complication [49, 50]. Increased oxidative stress (OS) is a key contributor to HG-induced diabetic damages [51]. Increased OS is a possible biochemical mechanism linking the onset of DM and its complications due to OS [52–54]. Furthermore, hypertrophy and myocardial fibrosis are also associated with endothelial cell dysfunction (ECD), inflammation and abnormal vascular remodelling seen in DCM [45]. The activation of endothelial cells (ECs) from a quiescent phenotype to vasoconstriction, pro-inflammatory and pro-apoptotic state can also result in ECD [55]. The exposure of the blood vessels to high fluctuating levels of elevated blood glucose (HG) is a known factor for ECD [56].

An increase in myocardial stiffness is an early sign in the pathogenesis of DCM. This increase in myocardial tissue stiffness is a result of increased collagen production by fibroblasts along with the fibrotic replacement of apoptotic/necrotic cells [57]. Collagen type I and type III fibres accumulate in the epicardial (EPI) layer of the heart and perivascular domains, whereas type IV is mostly found in the endocardial (ENDO) layer of the myocardium [58]. The increased stiffness in diabetic hearts may be due to an increase in the stiffness of cardiac myocytes within the myocardium. Although the changes in stiffness are not dramatic, they may be enough to cause or to contribute to increased cardiac workload over time, leading to DCM progression [59]. At the molecular level, DCM leads to prolongation and enhanced temporal dispersion of the repolarization phase of cardiac action potential (CAP) in myocytes leading to alterations of the spatial heterogeneity of ion channel expression and AP duration [60]. The major recognised factors of DCM are insulin resistance (IR) and hyperinsulinemia [61]. A disruption of insulin-mediated glucose metabolism occurs during IR and hyperinsulinemia which can significantly alter the efficiency of metabolism in cardiac muscle as well as skeletal muscle. The diabetic heart is affected by insulin in both systematic metabolism abnormalities via direct effects on insulin signalling pathways in the myocardium [62]. The early recognised change in insulin resistance in the heart is the impaired ability of insulin to increase glucose transport [63]. Recently, it was found that IR is linked to cardiac contractile dysfunction. In addition, a previous study, has developed a new IR rat model in which the animals were fed on a high cholesterol fructose (HCF) diet [63]. These results demonstrate that IR is directly linked to biochemical changes in the heart, thereby contributing to the development of DCM. Despite the recent advances in this field, our understanding of the initiation and progress of DCM is still very limited.

7. Conclusion

CVDs are considered as the leading cause of deaths globally and they are multifactorial in nature affecting the heart, the blood vessels and the blood. The flow diagram in **Figure 1** reveals the processes and mechanism(s) whereby diabetes-induced elevated hyperglycemia, hyperinsulinemia and hyperlipidemia can lead to oxidative stress, inflammation, mitochondrial dysfunction and other mechanisms, all resulting in cardiac dysfunction, including HF, DCM ,arrhythmias and sudden cardiac death., Initially, these dysfunctions are induced at the cellular, sub-cellular and molecular levels in the heart and they include changes in size, shape and function of the myocardium, including cellular calcium homeostasis. If the heart is left untreated, then it can develop, hypertrophy and disarray of the myofilaments and subsequently apoptosis and infiltration of fibrosis leading to remodeling of the myocardium. Moreover, chronic inflammation associated with cardiac dysfunction

DOI: http://dx.doi.org/10.5772/intechopen.88149

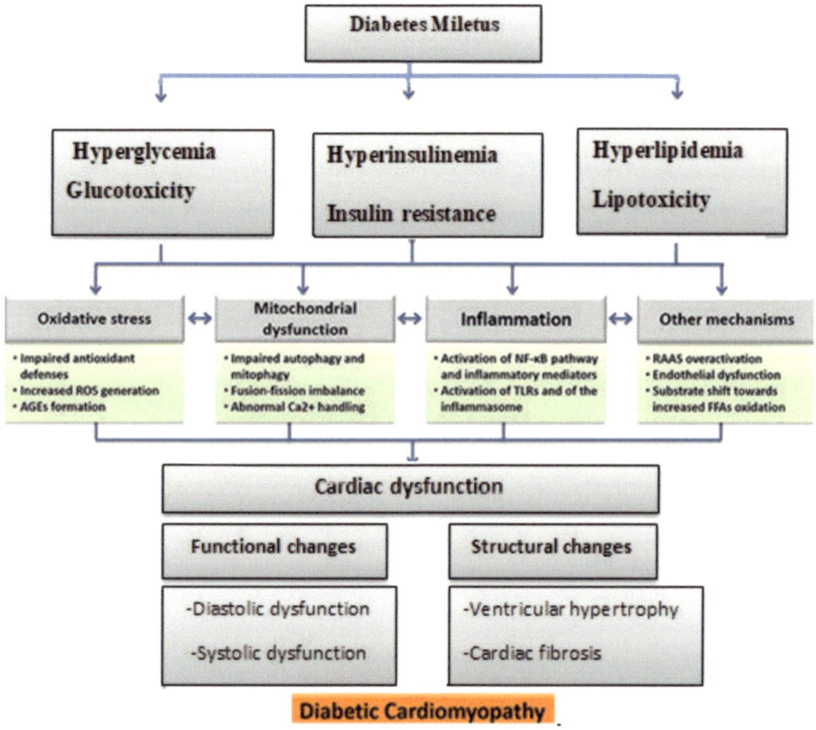

Figure 1.
Changes occurring in the heart during diabetic cardiomyopathy. DCM in turn can lead to structural and functional changes at cellular and subcellular levels in the myocardium.

can also result in damage and subsequent failure to a number of organs in the body including the heart and kidneys where the dynamics of blood flow is disturbed. In relation to the myocardium, there is an increase in CAPD and subsequently elevated diastolic [Ca^{2+}]. The end-result is a delay in contraction and blood ejection from the heart. This leads to slower relaxation and filling process in the heart. Over time, the whole process will lead to a weak heart or DCM and subsequently, death of the patient. The cellular and molecular mechanisms associated with chronic inflammation and the cardiovascular system are not fully known and the literature suggests the need for further research into novel inflammatory markers of CVD risk.

Author details

Manal M.A. Smail[1,2], Chris F. Howarth[1], Jaipaul Singh[3*] and Abla Mohamed Ismail[4]

1 Department of Physiology, College of Medicine and Health Sciences, United Arab Emirates University, United Arab Emirates

2 Fatima College for Health Sciences, United Arab Emirates

3 School of Forensic and Applied Sciences, University of Central Lancashire, Preston, Lancashire, England, United Kingdom

4 Corniche Hospital, United Arab Emirates

*Address all correspondence to: jsingh3@uclan.ac.uk

IntechOpen

© 2019 The Author(s). Licensee IntechOpen. This chapter is distributed under the terms of the Creative Commons Attribution License (http://creativecommons.org/licenses/by/3.0), which permits unrestricted use, distribution, and reproduction in any medium, provided the original work is properly cited.

References

[1] Kannel WB, McGee DL. Diabetes and cardiovascular disease: The Framingham study. The Journal of the American Medical Association. 1979;**241**(19):2035-2038

[2] Roger VL. The heart failure epidemic. International Journal of Environmental Research and Public Health. 2010;**7**(4):1807-1830

[3] Willerson JT, Ridker PM. Inflammation as a cardiovascular risk factor. Circulation. 2004;**109**(2):10

[4] Bastard JP, Maachi M, Lagathu C, Kim MJ, Caron M, Vidal H, et al. Recent advances in the relationship between obesity, inflammation, and insulin resistance. European Cytokine Network. 2006;**17**(1):4-12

[5] Mendis S, Puska P, Norrving B. Global Atlas on Cardiovascular Disease Prevention and Control. World Health Organization; 2011

[6] Moran AE, Forouzanfar MH, Roth GA, Ezzati M, Flaxman A. The global burden of ischemic heart disease in 1990 and 2010: The global burden of disease 2010 study. Circulation. 2014;**129**(14):245-254

[7] Belal AM. Nutrition-related chronic diseases epidemic in UAE: Can we stand to stop it? Sudanese Journal of Public Health. 2009;**4**:383-392

[8] Zimmet P, Alberti KG, Shaw J. Global and societal implications of the diabetes epidemic. Nature. 2001;**414**(6865):782-787

[9] Lockhart MM, Phelp AL, Van den Hoff MJB, Wessels A. The epicardium and the development of the atrioventricular junction in the murine heart. Developmental Biology. 2014;**2**:1-17

[10] Parashar K, Starling SK. Diabetes: History and traditional medication. Scientific Research. 2015;**4**(9):337-342

[11] Alcoholism, heart failure and diabetes (clinical conference). Medicina (Buenos Aires). 1993;**53**(3):239-247

[12] Houser SR. Role of RyR2 phosphorylation in heart failure and arrhythmias: Protein kinase A-mediated hyperphosphorylation of the ryanodine receptor at serine 2808 does not alter cardiac contractility or cause heart failure and arrhythmias. Circulation Research. 2014;**114**(8):1320-1327

[13] Hasenfuss G. Alterations of calcium-regulatory proteins in heart failure. Cardiovascular Research. 2016;**37**(2):279-289

[14] Houser SR, Marguiles KB. Is depressed myocyte contractility centrally involved in heart failure? Circulation Research. 2016;**92**(4):350-358

[15] Mann DL, Bristow MR. Mechanisms and models in heart failure: The biomechanical model and beyond. Circulation. 2005;**111**(21):2837-3849

[16] Pieske B, Maier LS, Piacentino V III, Weisser J, Hasenfuss G, Houser SR. Rate dependence of [Na+]i and contractility in nonfailing and failing human myocardium. Circulation. 2002;**106**(4):447-453

[17] Scrutinio D, Napoli V, Passantino A, Ricci A, Lagioia R, Rizzon P. Low-dose dobutamine responsiveness in idiopathic dilated cardiomyopathy: Relation to exercise capacity and clinical outcome. European Heart Journal. 2000;**21**(11):927-934

[18] Cohn JN, Johnson G, Ziesche S, Cobb F, Francis G, Tristani F, et al. A comparison of enalapril with

hydralazine-isosorbide dinitrate in the treatment of chronic congestive heart failure. The New England Journal of Medicine. 1991;**325**(5):303-310

[19] Swynghedauw B. Molecular mechanisms of myocardial remodeling. Physiological Reviews. 1999;**79**(1):215-262

[20] Spinas E, Kritas SK, Saggini A, Mobili A, Antinolfi P, Pantalone A. Role of mast cells in atherosclerosis: A classical inflammatory disease. Immunopharmacology. 2014;**27**:517-521

[21] Tsoupras AB, Iatrou C, Frangia C, Demopoulos CA. The implication of platelet-activating factor in cancer growth and metastasis: Potent beneficial role of PAF-inhibitors and antioxidants. Infectious Disorders Drug Targets. 2009;**9**:390-399

[22] Tsoupras A, Lordan R, Zabetakis I. Inflammation, not cholesterol, is a cause of chronic disease. Nutrients. 2018;**10**(5):1-38

[23] Galkina E, Ley K. Immune and inflammatory mechanisms of atherosclerosis. Annual Review of Immunology. 2009;**27**:165-197

[24] Libby P, Hansson GK. Inflammation and immunity in diseases of the arterial tree: Players and layers. Circulation. 2015;**116**:307-311

[25] Welsh P, Grassia G, Botha S, Sattar N. Targeting inflammation to reduce cardiovascular disease risk: A realistic clinical prospect? British Journal of Pharmacology. 2017;**174**(22):3898-3913

[26] Ezzati M. Contributions of risk factors and medical care to cardiovascular mortality trends. Nature Reviews. Cardiology. 2015;**12**:508-530

[27] Badran MLI, Type II. Diabetes mellitus in Arabic-speaking countries. International Journal of Endocrinology. 2012;**8**:1-11

[28] Hypertension control: Report of a WHO expert committee. World Health Organization Technical Report Series. 1996;**862**:1-83

[29] Olivetti G, Ricci R, Anversa P. Hyperplasia of myocyte nuclei in long-term cardiac hypertrophy in rats. The Journal of Clinical Investigation. 1987;**80**(6):1818-1821

[30] Pluim BM, Zwinderman AH, van der Laarse A, van der Wall EE. The athlete's heart. A meta-analysis of cardiac structure and function. Circulation. 2000;**101**:336-344

[31] Bansal N. Prediabetes diagnosis and treatment: A review. World Journal of Diabetes. 2015;**6**(2):296-303

[32] Ganz P, Braunwald E. Coronary Blood Flow and Myocardial Ischemia Heart Disease: A Textbook of Cardiovascular Medicine. Philadelphia: WB Saunders; 1997. pp. 1161-1183

[33] Herdson PB, Sommers HM, Jennings RB. A comparative study of the fine structure of normal and ischemic dog myocardium with special reference to early changes following temporary occlusion of a coronary artery. The American Journal of Pathology. 1965;**46**(3):367-386

[34] Tennant R, Wiggers CJ. The effect of coronary occlusion on myocardial contraction. The American Journal of Physiology. 1935;**112**(2):351-361

[35] Ferdinandy P, Schulz R, Baxter GF. Interaction of cardiovascular risk factors with myocardial ischemia/reperfusion injury, preconditioning, and postconditioning. Pharmacological Reviews. 2007;**59**(4):418-458

[36] Boudina S, Abel ED. Diabetic cardiomyopathy revisited. Circulation. 2007;**115**(25):3213-3223

[37] Kenchaiah S, Vasan RS. Heart failure in women-insights from

the Framingham heart study. Cardiovascular Drugs and Therapy. 2015;**29**(4):377-390

[38] Voulgari C, Papadogiannis D, Tentolouris N. Diabetic cardiomyopathy: From the pathophysiology of the cardiac myocytes to current diagnosis and management strategies. Vascular Health and Risk Management. 2010;**21**(6):883-903

[39] Bell DS. Diabetic cardiomyopathy. A unique entity or a complication of coronary artery disease? Diabetes Care. 1995;**18**(5):708-714

[40] Aragno M, Mastrocola R, Medana C, Catalano MG, Vercellinatto I, Danni O, et al. Oxidative stress-dependent impairment of cardiac-specific transcription factors in experimental diabetes. Endocrinology. 2006;**147**(12):5967-5974

[41] Asbun J, Villarreal FJ. The pathogenesis of myocardial fibrosis in the setting of diabetic cardiomyopathy. Journal of the American College of Cardiology. 2006;**47**(4):693-700

[42] Poornima IG, Parikh P, Shannon RP. Diabetic cardiomyopathy: The search for a unifying hypothesis. Circulation Research. 2006;**98**(5):596-605

[43] Jia G, Demarco VG, Sowers JR. Insulin resistance and hyperinsulinaemia in diabetic cardiomyopathy. Nature Reviews Endocrinology. 2016;**12**(3):144-153

[44] Adeghate E. Molecular and cellular basis of the aetiology and management of diabetic cardiomyopathy: A short review. Molecular and Cellular Biochemistry. 2004;**261**(1-2):187-191

[45] Boudina S, Abel ED. Diabetic cardiomyopathy, causes and effects. Reviews in Endocrine & Metabolic Disorders. 2010;**11**(1):31-39

[46] Brownlee M. The pathobiology of diabetic complications: A unifying mechanism. Diabetes. 2005;**54**:1615-1625

[47] Berg TJ, Snorgaard O, Faber J, Torjesen PA, Hildebrandt P, Mehlsen J, et al. Serum levels of advanced glycation end products are associated with left ventricular diastolic function in patients with type 1 diabetes. Diabetes Care. 1999;**22**(7):1186-1190

[48] Grundy SM, Benjamin IJ, Burke GL, Chait A, Eckel RH, Howard BV, et al. Diabetes and cardiovascular disease: A statement for healthcare professionals from the American Heart Association. Circulation. 1999;**100**(10):1134-1146

[49] Francis GS. Diabetic cardiomyopathy: Fact or fiction? Heart. 2001;**85**(3):247-248

[50] Sowers JR, Epstein M, Frohlich ED. Diabetes, hypertension, and cardiovascular disease: An update. Hypertension. 2001;**37**:1053-1059

[51] Poirier P, Bogaty P, Philippon F, Garneau C, Fortin C. Diastolic dysfunction in normotensive men with well-controlled type 2 diabetes: Importance of manoeuvres in echocardiographic screening for preclinical diabetic cardiomyopathy. Diabetes Care. 2001;**24**:5-10

[52] Giardino I, Fard AK, Hatchell DL, Brownlee M. Aminoguanidine inhibits reactive oxygen species formation, lipid peroxidation, and oxidant-induced apoptosis. Diabetes. 1998;**47**(7):1114-1120

[53] Costa MA, Balaszczuk AM, Dominguez A, Catanzaro O, Arranz C. Effects of L-NAME and L-Arg on arterial blood pressure in normotensive and hypertensive streptozotocin

diabetic rats. Acta Physiologica, Pharmacologica et Therapeutica Latinoamericana. 1998;**48**(2):59-63

[54] Cai L, Kang YJ. Oxidative stress and diabetic cardiomyopathy: A brief review. Cardiovascular Toxicology. 2001;**1**:181-193

[55] Xu J, Zou MH. Molecular insights and therapeutic targets for diabetic endothelial dysfunction. Circulation. 2009;**120**:1266-1286

[56] Hadi HA, Suwaidi JA. Endothelial dysfunction in diabetes mellitus. Vascular Health and Risk Management. 2007;**3**:853-876

[57] Tang M, Zhang W, Jiang H, Dai H, Zhang Y. High glucose promotes the production of collagen types I and III by cardiac fibroblasts through a pathway dependent on extracellular-signal-regulated kinase 1/2. Molecular and Cellular Biochemistry. 2007;**301**(1):109-114

[58] Kajstura J, Fiordaliso F, Andreoli AM, Li B, Chimenti S, Medow MS, et al. IGF-1 overexpression inhibits the development of diabetic cardiomyopathy and angiotensin II-mediated oxidative stress. Diabetes. 2001;**50**(6):1414-1424

[59] Michaelson J, Hariharan V, Huang H. Hyperglycemic and hyperlipidemic conditions alter cardiac cell biomechanical properties. Biophysical Journal. 2014;**106**(11):2322-2329

[60] Okin PM, Devereux RB, Lee ET, Galloway JM, Howard BV. Electrocardiographic repolarization complexity and abnormality predict all-cause and cardiovascular mortality in diabetes: The strong heart study. Diabetes. 2004;**53**(2):434-440

[61] Despres JP, Lamarche B, Mauriege P, Cantin B, Dagenais GR, Moorjani S, et al. Hyperinsulinemia as an independent risk factor for ischemic heart disease [see comments]. The New England Journal of Medicine. 1996;**334**(15):952-957

[62] Huang JP, Huang LM. Insulin Resistance and Cardiomyopathy, Cardiomyopathies. Taiwan: Chang Gung University; 2012

[63] Wright JJ, Kim J, Buchanan J, Boudina S, Sena S, Bakirtzi K, et al. Mechanisms for increased myocardial fatty acid utilization following short-term high-fat feeding. Cardiovascular Research. 2009;**82**(2):351-360

Chapter 8

Peripartum Cardiomyopathy: Facts and Figures

Nissar Shaikh, Firdos Ummunnisa, Arshad Chanda, Mohammad A. Imran, Adel Ganaw, Umm-e-Amara, Zia Mahmood, M.A. Rahman, Mohammad Nayeemuddin, Moad Ehfeda, Muhammad Zubair, Ahmed Atef Shible, Ranjan Matthias, Muhammad Shakeel Riaz, Hafiz Hamid Habib, Masood Khattak and A.R. Raju Vegesna

Abstract

Peripartum cardiomyopathy (PPCM) is a rare clinical entity during pregnancy. PPCM is a diagnosis of exclusion. These patients do not have prior history of heart disease, and there are no other known possible causes of heart failure. It is more common in African countries, may be related to the consumption of kanwa, in the postpartum period. The multiparity, African descent and pregnancy-induced hypertension are a few risk factors for PPCM. The exact etiology of PPCM is not known; possible theories range from myocarditis to the maladaptation to the changes of pregnancy. The clinical manifestation varies from shortness of breath to thromboembolic phenomenon. Echocardiography is essential for diagnosis as well as differential diagnosis of PPCM. These patients preferably are managed in tertiary healthcare facilities. Anticoagulation and antiarrhythmic medications are pillars for the management of PPCM patients. If required, mechanical devices should be used temporarily. PPCM patients may need heart transplant. The beneficial role of bromocriptine and immunosuppression is not clear in PPCM patients. Subsequent pregnancies should be avoided to prevent the PPCM occurrence.

Keywords: echocardiography, left ventricular ejection fraction, peripartum cardiomyopathy, multiparity, heart failure, anticoagulation and antiarrhythmic medications

1. Introduction

Peripartum cardiomyopathy (PPCM) is the heart muscle weakness that begins during the late pregnancy and extending into 5 months in puerperium without any other known etiology. PPCM is a dilated cardiomyopathy and involves systolic dysfunction, decreased left ventricular ejection fraction (EF), and congestive heart failure. There is an increased risk of atrial and ventricular arrhythmias and thromboembolism. PPCM is a diagnosis of exclusion, patients have no prior history of heart disease, and there are no other known possible causes of heart failure (HF). Echocardiogram is essentially used for both diagnosis and monitoring purposes in the progress of PPCM. Although initially described in the 18th century, it was recognized as distinct clinical in 1930, and Demakis et al. described and defined PPCM [1]. PPCM was initially termed as pregnancy-associated cardiomyopathy, toxic postpartum heart failure, Meadows' syndrome, postpartum myocarditis, and Zaria syndrome.

2. Definition

There are varieties of definitions for PPCM; the more simplified one is by the working group on peripartum cardiomyopathy from the European Society of Cardiology in 2010. It avoids under diagnosis by adopting a broader definition. It contains the following characteristics:

1. The development of heart failure in last month of pregnancy or up to 5 months in postpartum period

2. Absence of another known or identifiable cause for heart failure

3. Systolic dysfunction of left ventricle (LV) and LV ejection fraction of less than 0.45 with or without LV dilatation [2]

3. Epidemiology

PPCM constitutes less than 1% of all cardiovascular events related to pregnancy. It is more common in Africa, 1:300 pregnancies. This may be due to the consumption of kanwa, a tradition, for 40 postpartum days. Kanwa is a dry salt and causes hypervolemia and hypertension. Ninety percent of PPCM occurs within 2 months of delivery [3]. In a recently concluded study about the incidence of PPCM from 43 countries, affecting females from all ethnicity and all continents, the incidence widely differs depending on geographic location. PPCM was common in Nigeria (1100), Haiti (1300), South Africa (11,000), Canada (12,400), and Denmark (110,149) and was lowest in Japan (1,20,000 live births). There are case reports from other countries [4]. Hence the information is not complete as many countries are not having a registry. The higher incidence in Nigeria may be related to abovementioned postpartum high salt intake or may be a genetic factor superimposing the geographic and dietary variabilities [5].

4. Risk factors

The following are the risk factors for PCCM, even though the etiology of PPCM is still not clear.

1. Age over 30 years, pregnancy with multiple fetuses [6].

2. Multiparty, African descent [7].

3. Maternal cocaine abuse [8].

4. Long-term tocolytic therapy [9].

5. History of preeclampsia, eclampsia, or peripartum hypertension, the hypertensive disorders of pregnancy are significant predispose for PPCM, and the preeclampsia patient is four times more susceptible for developing PPCM [10].

5. Etiopathology

In the pathology of peripartum cardiomyopathy, the macroscopic view is a pale myocardium, dilated heart often with intramural thrombus in the ventricles. There will be endocardial thickening and pericardial effusion. The myocardial cellular hypertrophy and myofibril degeneration with areas of fibrosis with interstitial edema are the nonspecific findings. In a small group of patients, there are features of myocarditis with the presence of inflammatory cell infiltration of myocardium, focal necrosis, variable hypertrophy, and fibrosis of the myocardium [11].

Although PPCM is a separate clinical entity, the exact etiology of PPCM is still not known. Following hypothesis had been proposed for the etiology.

5.1 Familial

The familial clustering of PPCM is well known; it could be due to genetic or environmental factors. Ancestry with African genomics may be a risk factor and explains the higher prevalence of PPCM in Haiti, Africa, and black women in other countries. The guanine nucleotide-binding protein beta-3 (GNB3) subunit has a polymorphism called C825T. This polymorphism is associated with an increased risk of hypertension, low plasma renin, and cardiac remodeling. GNB3 has a prevalence of 50% in black individuals compared with 10% in white individuals [12].

5.2 Myocarditis

First time Melvin et al. proposed myocarditis as a cause for PPCM. Myocarditis could be viral or autoimmune. With pregnancy there is increased in susceptibility to both. In another study, endomyocardial biopsies in five patients showed features of myocarditis. The reason for lesser positive biopsy report among the studies may be related to small sample size and timing of biopsy with relation to the onset of symptoms. The incidence of inflammation is greater in patients who are biopsied soon after presentation [13, 14]. The proinflammatory-inflammatory cytokines may play a role in the pathogenesis and progression of PPCM, as the cytokines that are elevated in PPCM compared with controls include tumor necrosis factor (TNF)-alpha and interleukin-6 [15].

5.3 Abnormal immune response

The entrance of fetal cells into the maternal circulation remains in the circulation without rejection due to weak immunogenic paternal haplotype of chorionic cell. If these cells lodge into the cardiac tissue, immune response may be triggered. The raised titres of immunoglobulins and other autoantibodies in patients with PPCM are suggestive of abnormal immune response, whereas other studies found no significant difference in levels of immunoglobulins and other autoantibodies in PPCM and control group of patients [12, 16].

5.4 Maladaptation to stress of pregnancy

The hyperdynamic circulation during pregnancy causes remodeling and transient hypertrophy of the left ventricle. The exaggerated reduction in left ventricular systolic function with stress of gestational hypertension may contribute to heart failure in PPCM patients. In pregnancy 40–50% increase in blood volume and cardiac output occurs which results in transient LV hypertrophy. The hemodynamic stress of gestational hypertension, may contribute to the development of PPCM and heart failure, with an angiogenic imbalance may better explain the association between preeclampsia and PPCM [17].

5.5 Angiogenic imbalance and balance

Human and animal studies suggest that PPCM is caused by systemic angiogenic imbalance. Animals that lack cardiac PGC-1α, a regulator of proangiogenic factors such as VEGF, develop severe PPCM. These data may also explain why preeclampsia and multiple gestations are risk factors for PPCM. During late gestation, the human placenta secretes VEGF inhibitors such as soluble fms-like tyrosine kinase 1 (sFlt1), which damages the vasculature, with higher levels seen with multiple gestations or preeclampsia. Preeclampsia and multiple gestations are risk factors for PPCM as in these patients subclinical cardiac dysfunction correlates with sFlt1 levels [18].

5.6 Prolactin role

Alteration in prolactin processing is involved in the pathogenesis of peripartum cardiomyopathy; animal with a knockout in the cardiac tissue-specific signal

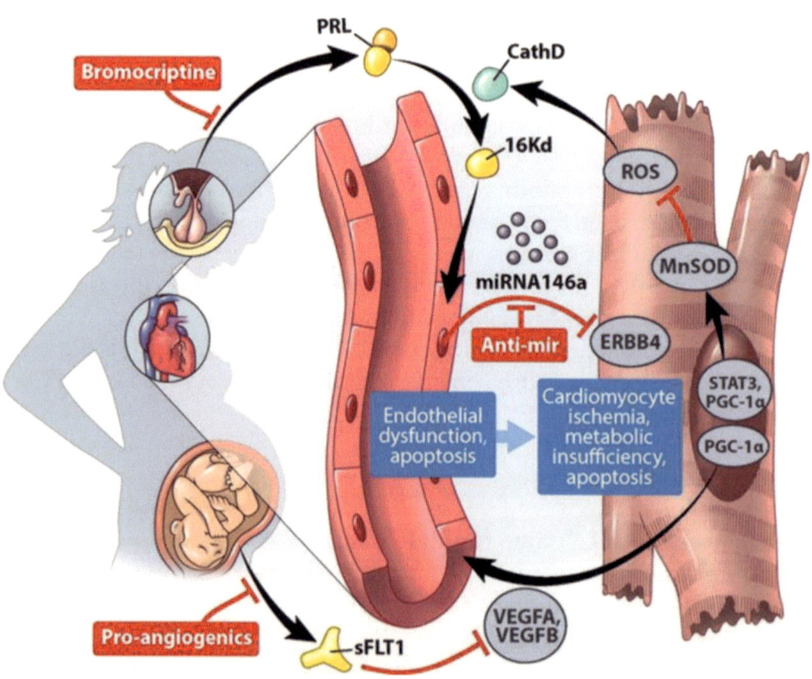

Figure 1.
Summary of etiopathogenesis of PPCM (from [19]).

transduction and activator of transcription 3 (STAT3) developed PPCM. Reduction in STAT3 leads to increased cleavage of prolactin into an anti-angiogenic and proapoptotic 16 kDa isoform by cathepsin D. The 16 kDa prolactin fragment (16K PRL) causes endothelial damage leading to myocardial dysfunction; 16K PRL induces microRNA-146a expression in endothelial cells, which leads to most of the anti-angiogenic effects of 16K PRL. Females with PPCM have elevated levels of microRNA-146a compared with healthy postpartum women or women with other cardiomyopathies (**Figure 1**) [20].

6. Clinical presentations

PPCM is common in first postpartum month; it is also rare before 36 weeks of gestation (**Figure 2**). The common presentations of PPCM are dyspnea, cough, orthopnea, and paroxysmal nocturnal dyspnea, which may be confused with the physiological changes of pregnancy. Initial diagnosis may be delayed since symptoms such as nonspecific fatigue, shortness of breath, and pedal edema are similar to those observed in normal pregnancy The patient may have arrhythmia and even cardiac arrest rarely [4]; PPCM can present with thromboembolic manifestations; patients with left ventricular ejection fraction (LVEF) < 35% are at risk for developing left ventricular thrombus. PPCM is manifested after 38 weeks of pregnancy, whereas pregnant patients with chronic heart disease develop sign and symptoms of heart failure in the second trimester of pregnancy due to stress of hemodynamic overload.

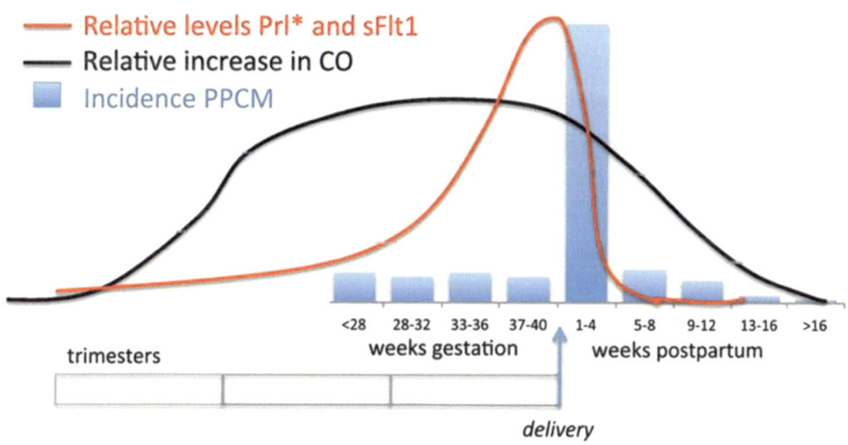

Figure 2.
Pregnancy and occurrence of PPCM [19].

7. Signs and symptoms

Signs and symptoms are variable and similar to that in other forms of systolic HF due to cardiomyopathy. Signs include an elevated jugular venous pressure, displaced apical impulse, a third heart sound, and a murmur of mitral regurgitation. Signs and symptoms of systemic or pulmonary thromboembolism may be present. Various studies have reported varying rates of thromboembolism, and further data are required to quantify the risk of this complication. Patients with PPCM left ventricular thrombus were identified by echocardiography in 16 of 100 patients with PPCM (with mean LVEF of 26%) in a case series [2, 21].

8. Diagnosis

As mentioned initially diagnosis of PPCM based on three clinical criteria, development of heart failure in last month of pregnancy or in the initial 5 months following delivery with the absence of another identifiable cause of HF and left ventricular (LV) systolic dysfunction with an left ventricular ejection fraction (LVEF) of < 45%. The last criteria will exclude patients with accelerated hypertension, diastolic dysfunction, systemic infection, pulmonary embolism, or preeclampsia or amniotic fluid embolus. Chest X-ray, electrocardiogram (ECG), and echocardiogram should be performed in patients who are clinically suspected of having PPCM.

Studies showed brain natriuretic peptide (BNP) levels, cardiac magnetic resonance (CMR) imaging, cardiac catheterization, and endomyocardial biopsy (EMB) will be helpful in these patients. Bacterial cultures and viral titers are usually not indicated, as these tests are nonspecific and without proven value in patients with myocarditis. The novel markers, plasma concentrations of proangiogenic and antiangiogenic factors, placenta growth factor, and fms-like tyrosine kinase 1 receptor, have been proposed to be used to distinguish patients with PPCM [22].

8.1 Electrocardiogram (ECG)

It is not specific in PPCM patients and may show sinus tachycardia rarely arrhythmias and nonspecific ST segment and T wave changes. PR and QRS intervals may be prolonged. An ECG is helpful in identifying conditions in the differential diagnosis such as myocardial infarction and pulmonary embolism [1].

8.2 Brain natriuretic peptide (BNP)

Plasma BNP or pro-BNP (proBNP) measurement is helpful in the evaluation and diagnosis of patients with heart failure. Patients with PPCM have increased BNP and NT-proBNP levels, higher than seen in healthy women during pregnancy or postpartum.

8.3 Chest X-rays

Commonly it will show enlargement of the cardiac silhouette with pulmonary congestion and/or interstitial edema and pleural effusions. However, a chest radiograph is not necessary to make a diagnosis of HF or PPCM and exposes the patient to ionizing radiation.

8.4 Echocardiography (echo)

Echocardiogram is essential in the diagnosis of PPCM; it reveals a global reduction in LV systolic function with LVEF of < 45%. Left ventricle is commonly but not always dilated. Assessment of right ventricular systolic pressures can be performed (**Figure 3**). Echo may show presence of left atrial thrombus, dilated right ventricle, abnormal ventricular wall motion, mitral and tricuspid regurgitation, and pericardial effusion.

8.5 Cardiac magnetic resonance imaging (CMR)

If echocardiography is technically suboptimal, CMR can help. It helps in assessing LV function and LV volumes. Experience with CMR in PPCM is limited and its role is still being evaluated.

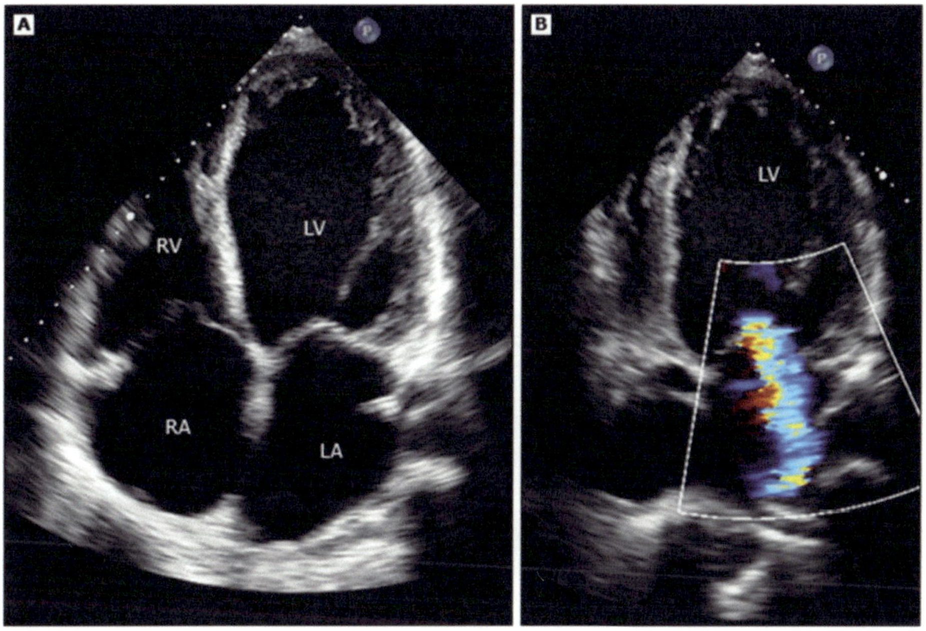

Figure 3.
Four chamber view of PPCM A: Echocardiographic four chamber view of PPCM. B: Echocardiogrhic Mitral regurgitation view of PPCM.

8.6 Cardiac catheterization

It may be helpful in critically ill patients, requiring a complete assessment or ongoing evaluation of their hemodynamic state.

8.7 Left heart catheterization and coronary angiography

It is required in selected patients in whom it is necessary to evaluate coronary artery disease as a potential cause for the cardiomyopathy. The coronary angiography exposes the patient to ionizing radiation and it is commonly not required in patients with suspected PPCM.

8.8 Endomyocardial biopsy (EMB)

EMB is recommended in clinical scenarios in which a biopsy is anticipated to yield a diagnosis of a specific condition with treatment implications. These scenarios include heart failure with hemodynamic compromise of less than 2 weeks duration or heart failure of less than 3 months duration if associated with heart block, new ventricular arrhythmias, or refractory heart failure. EMB is not recommended for the routine evaluation of heart failure, as there are no pathognomonic findings in PPCM. The risk of a serious acute complication is less than 1% using flexible bioptomes.

9. Differential diagnosis

PPCM should be differentiated from other forms of cardiomyopathy (**Figure 4**), heart failure, pulmonary thromboembolism, severe eclampsia, and pneumonia. From history, in physical examination and investigations, one must exclude myocardial infarction, idiopathic dilated cardiomyopathy, and valvular heart disease [9].

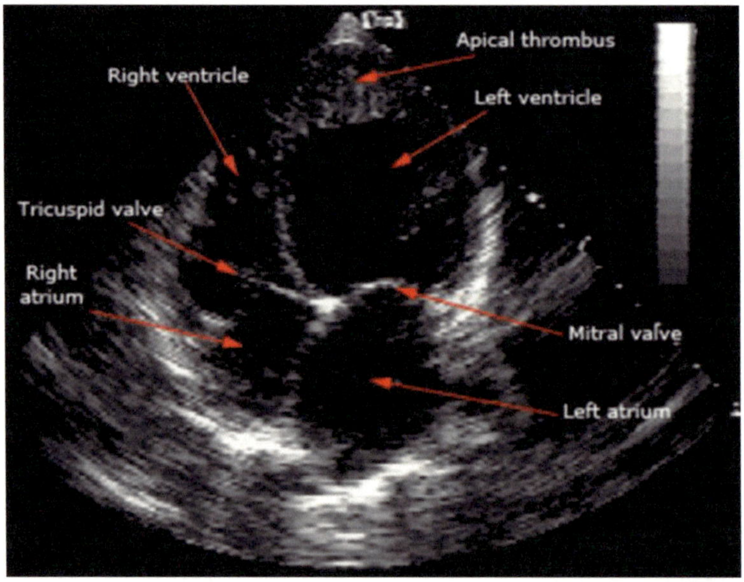

Figure 4.
Four chamber echocardiographic view showing thrombus in PPCM.

10. Management

The therapeutic approach of PPCM is the same as for other types of HF with left ventricular systolic dysfunction. Precautions should be taken to ensure the safety of the mother and the unborn or breastfeeding child; these patients may need antiarrhythmic drugs, anticoagulation therapy, mechanical support, and the use of investigational medications (bromocriptine).

The cornerstone in the management of PPCM is to reduce preload and after load and increase the cardiac contractility. Heart failure during pregnancy may be acute or acute on chronic. The pregnant patient with known cardiac disease can present in stable condition during early stages of pregnancy. Careful physical examination should be done. Their management is mainly adjustment of their medication and monitoring for cardiac failure. The initial New York Heart Association functional class status should be documented. Serial ECG and echocardiogram should be performed.

Patients presenting heart failure during pregnancy or the peripartum period require a detail history and physical examination and the evaluation of severity of decompensation. An ECG may reveal deteriorating left ventricular functions, arrhythmia, LVH, or arterial abnormality. The therapeutic approach in these patients includes optimizing hemodynamics, reducing after load, optimizing preload, and cardiac contractility. These can be achieved by treatment of pulmonary congestion, control of hyper-/hypotension, treatment of cardiac arrhythmia, and prevention of thromboembolic events.

10.1 Antiarrhythmic therapy

Arrhythmias are common in patients hospitalized for PPCM. The occurrence of arterial and ventricular arrhythmias is variable. In one of the studies, 18.7% PPCM patients had an arrhythmia, and ventricular tachycardia was in 4.2% with cardiac arrest in 2.2%. In smaller studies, the reported incidence of ventricular tachycardia was 20 and 25%. The atrial fibrillation was reported to occur in 3.1–11.9% of patients with PPCM [23].

Ventricular arrhythmias should be treated aggressively in PPCM patients. Class III antiarrythmic medications are the best option. Intravenous medications are needed in PPCM patients admitted to the intensive care therapy unit. Therapy with inotropes such as dobutamine, adrenaline, and milrinone should be directed by invasive cardiac monitoring. While interpreting the invasive hemodynamic monitoring, one should take into account the normal changes that occur during pregnancy. Digoxin is safe to use in pregnancy. Diuretics can be used if salt restriction is not sufficient. Beta-blocker improves left ventricular function in patients of PPCM, but ACE inhibitors are the drugs of choice in postpartum PPCM [24].

10.2 Anticoagulation therapy

The anticoagulation in PPCM is a must as pregnancy itself is a hypercoagulable state, in addition to PPCM, dilatation of heart, and turbulent flow of blood. For pregnant patients requiring anticoagulation, decisions and choosing anticoagulation therapy are challenging due to the risk of bleeding in all stages of pregnancy and the potential teratogenic effects of warfarin in the first trimester, dosage of various agents, and management during labor and delivery. PPCM patients receiving bromocriptine have an increased risk of thromboembolic events; hence, it is suggested to start anticoagulation therapy in patients with PPCM treated with bromocriptine. There is no clear data, but expert suggests anticoagulation for patients with PPCM with acute cardiac thrombus or evidence of systemic embolism. Before delivery unfraction or low-molecular-weight heparin is the choice, whereas in postpartum period warfarin is used.

10.3 Mechanical and device support and cardiac transplantation

The decisions to use implantable cardioverter defibrillator (ICD) or cardiac resynchronization therapy in PPCM patients should be taken after a detailed natural history and the potential of recovery of ventricular function. All these therapies should be deferred at least for 3 months and possibly for 6 months of presentation as 20–60% of PPCM patients have complete recovery of left ventricular ejection functions to normal by 6 months to 5 years [25].

Mechanical circulatory support (MCS) is considered early for PPCM patients who are hemodynamically unstable and unresponsive to medical therapy with maximal inotropic support. A device can be implanted in the acute phase either to work as a bridge-to-recovery and subsequent weaning when the ventricular function improves, or it can be a bridge-to-bridge for implantation of a longer durable device. The bridge-to-transplantation is rarely required as the initial approach as a high proportion of PPCM patients will have recovery of ventricular function. Hence initially a temporary device should be used if required in these patients.

Severely reduced LVEF alone should not be an indication for the use of aggressive therapies (MCS and cardiac transplantation) in PPCM patients. If MCS is indicated, various devices can be used including intra-aortic balloon counterpulsation (IABP), venoarterial extracorporeal membrane oxygenation (ECMO), and LV assist device (LVAD). The choice of device will depend on the hemodynamic status of the patient and local availability and expertise. Venoarterial ECMO has been associated with an increase in prolactin levels, which may be detrimental in PPCM patients [26].

Loyaga-Rendon et al. reported that the PPCM patients who received durable mechanical circulatory support had better survival rate than that of females without PPCM with a survival rate of 83% in PPCM. These may be related to PPCM patients who were younger and had fewer comorbidities. The rates of myocardial function recovery were poor, 6% in the PPCM group and 2% in without PPCM [27].

According to the older literature, the transplantation was performed in up to one-third of PPCM patients, whereas the contemporary reports demonstrate that transplantation rates vary from 4 to 23% of patients [28]. Hence PPCM patients with significant LV systolic dysfunction should be managed at a tertiary center with transplant facilities.

In a large study, it is found that the long-term survival in transplanted PPCM patients was worse compared with all others undergoing transplantation. PPCM patient who received a cardiac transplant had higher mortality, higher incidence of rejection, poorer graft survival, and higher retransplantation rates. Younger patient age, higher allosensitization, higher pretransplant acuity, and increased rejection rates are all important factors for poorer outcomes in these PPCM patients [28].

10.3.1 Wearable cardioverter-defibrillators

Further multicenter trial would be valuable to establish if these devices are beneficial; in a single smaller study, it was found to be useful.

10.4 Medical investigational therapy

Following therapies are not recommended for PPCM patients as its efficacy and safety have not been established.

10.4.1 Bromocriptine

The use of bromocriptine therapy in PPCM patients is controversial. The preliminary data have shown a benefit of bromocriptine in PPCM patients, but further studies are needed to establish safety and efficacy; it is suggested not to routinely use bromocriptine in PPCM patients. Its use is based upon experimental animal studies of prevention of PPCM by prolactin blockade with bromocriptine. Smaller and observational reports showed the beneficial response to bromocriptine therapy in patients with PPCM [29].

A multicenter study showed that the rate of full recovery (LVEF $\geq$ 50%) was not significantly higher in the 8-week group compared with the 1-week group. The patients in this trial had better outcomes than observed in prior series, but a placebo control group was not included in the study [30]. One should start anticoagulation in PPCM patients treated with bromocriptine, as the risk of thromboembolic complications.

10.4.2 Immunosuppressive therapy

The advantage of immunosuppressive therapy has been found to be useful in PPCM patients with biopsy-proven myocarditis, but its efficacy is unclear, and empiric immunosuppression in the absence of evidence of a responsive form of myocarditis is not recommended [31]. These medications have significant side effects.

10.4.3 Intravenous immunoglobulin

This therapy is tried in patients with myocarditis or newly onset dilated cardiomyopathy with no clear evidence of clinical benefit, and the efficacy of this approach has not been confirmed in any type of myocarditis.

11. Delivery

In PPCM patient the risks and benefits of early delivery should be considered and discussed. The 2010 European Society of Cardiology working group statement advised that early delivery is not required if the maternal and fetal conditions are stable. But the patient-related factors, gestational age, cervical status, fetal status, and the potential cardiovascular impact of continuing pregnancy must be considered in timing delivery. The decisions regarding timing and mode of delivery should be based on combined multidisciplinary meeting. In PPCM patients with advanced heart failure, prompt delivery of fetus is indicated for maternal cardiovascular indications and hemodynamic instability. The elective cesarean delivery is preferred for PPCM patients with advanced heart failure requiring inotropic therapy or mechanical circulatory support [12].

12. Breastfeeding

According to the expert group, breastfeeding is to be avoided because of the potential effects of prolactin subfragments, but in a study where PPCM patients chose to breastfeed, none had adverse maternal effects, and that rate of recovery of left ventricular function was significantly higher in lactating women, and accordingly given the benefits of breastfeeding, it is recommended that women who are stable should continue breastfeeding as long as it is compatible with their heart failure medications [32].

13. Complications

The most common complication is thromboembolism. A premature delivery rate of 25% has been reported in cases with PPCM. PPCM cases had increased incidence of cesarean section up to 40% [33].

14. Prognosis

14.1 Maternal morbidity and mortality

The overall reported mortality rate in PPCM is better than other cardiomyopathy (**Figure 5**) patients approximately 10% in 2 years and 11–29% in 3 years [15]. Cardiac transplantation rates of less than 1–2% per year [15]. The mortality in PPCM patient is commonly caused by progressive pump failure, sudden death, or thromboembolic events. The following factors have been shown to increase the mortality in PPCCM patients (**Table 1**).

PPCM is associated with a significant morbidity including brain injury, cardiopulmonary arrest, fulminant pulmonary edema, thromboembolic complications, an-d defibrillator or pacemaker implantation [36].

14.2 Neonatal and obstetric outcomes

Lower section cesarean delivery was performed in 40% of patients, largely for obstetric indications. Preterm birth was noted in 25 and 5.9% of infants were small for date [37].

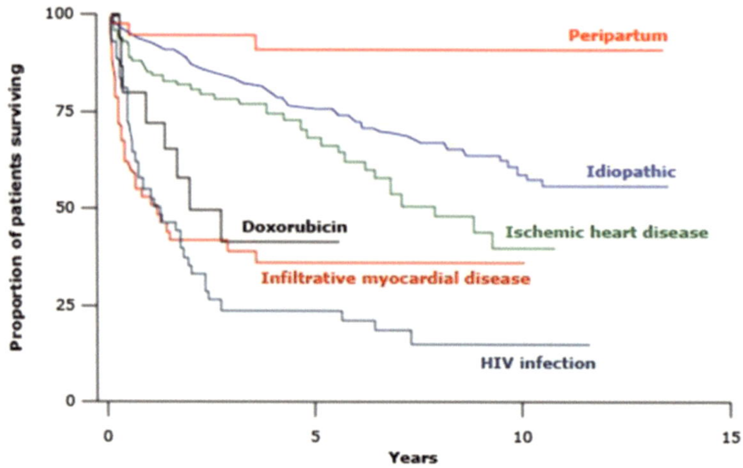

Figure 5.
Comparative mortality of cardiomyopathies [34].

Worse New York Heart Association functional class
Left ventricular ejection fraction (LVEF) ≤ 25%
Black race
Multiparity
Age more than 35 years [35]

Table 1.
Risk factors for increased mortality in PPCM.

14.3 Subsequent pregnancy

In patients who have recovered or not recovered from left ventricular failure due to PPCM, there is a high risk of PPCM in subsequent pregnancy. Termination of pregnancy may not prevent relapse.

15. Prevention

In patients who have recovered from left ventricular failure due to PPCM, there is a high risk of PPCM in subsequent pregnancy, and so the best way to avoid PPCM is avoid subsequent pregnancy. The literature suggests that the patient or her partner undergo a sterilization procedure or the patient use a highly effective non-estrogen method of contraception. Though the risk of recurrence appears to be less in PPCM patient with recovered LV function and LVEF > 25%, still these patients should receive counseling, including the option of avoidance of subsequent pregnancy due to the risk of relapse of PPCM, heart failure, and death. There is not much evidence on the safety of contraceptives in PPCM patients; it is advised that the estrogen-progestin contraceptives should be avoided in PPCM patients with persistent LV dysfunction because of their potential to increase the risk of thromboembolism [38].

16. Conclusion

PPCM is a rare but potentially life-threatening disease of pregnancy. PPCM is common in postpartum period. PPCM patient has various risk factor including hypertensive disorders of pregnancy. PPCM patients may present with shortness of breath, arrhythmias, pulmonary edema, and thromboembolic signs and symptoms. Echocardiography will essentially diagnose the PPCM, and it also helps in differential diagnosis. The management of PPCM patients is the management of heart failure with special consideration of fetus. Therapy may involve the use of mechanical devices or even cardiac transplant, but the anticoagulation and antiarrhythmic medication plays an important role in the management. The medical management with bromocriptine, immunosuppression, and immunoglobulin is controversial. Commonly the left ventricular function recovers, but in PCCM the maternal mortality is around 10%, and there is increased incidence of cesarean section. In subsequent pregnancy in patient with PCCM, heart failure may be more severe and may cause death. Family counseling is essential in these patients.

Author details

Nissar Shaikh[1*], Firdos Ummunnisa[2], Arshad Chanda[1], Mohammad A. Imran[1], Adel Ganaw[1], Umm-e-Amara[3], Zia Mahmood[1], M.A. Rahman[1], Mohammad Nayeemuddin[1], Moad Ehfeda[1], Muhammad Zubair[1], Ahmed Atef Shible[4], Ranjan Matthias[1], Muhammad Shakeel Riaz[1], Hafiz Hamid Habib[5], Masood Khattak[5] and A.R. Raju Vegesna[1]

1 Surgical Intensive Care, Hamad Medical Corporation, Doha, Qatar

2 Dr. Halima Al Tamimi, OBGY Center, Doha, Qatar

3 Apollo Medical College and Research Center, Hyderabad, India

4 Clinical Pharmacist, SICU, Hamad Medical Corporation, Doha, Qatar

5 Cardiology Department, Heart Hospital Hamad Medical Corporation, Doha, Qatar

*Address all correspondence to: nissatfirdous99@gmail.com

IntechOpen

© 2019 The Author(s). Licensee IntechOpen. This chapter is distributed under the terms of the Creative Commons Attribution License (http://creativecommons.org/licenses/by/3.0), which permits unrestricted use, distribution, and reproduction in any medium, provided the original work is properly cited.

References

[1] Demakis JG, Rahimtoola SH, Sutton GC, Meadows WR, Szanto PB, Tobin JR, et al. Natural course of peripartum cardiomyopathy. Circulation. 1971;**44**:1053-1061

[2] Sliwa K, Hilifiker-Kleiner D, Petrie MC, et al. Current state of knowledge on aetiology, diagnosis, management and therapy of peripartum cardiomyopathy: A position statement from the heart failure association of European society of cardiology working group on peripartum cardiomyopathy. European Journal of Heart Failure. 2010;**12**:767

[3] Shaikh N. An obstetric emergency called peripartum cardiomyopathy. Journal of Emergencies, Trauma, and Shock. 2010;**3**(1):39-42

[4] Raju V, Faraj JH, Shaikh N. Peripartum cardiomyopathy: Report of two cases and review of literature. Qatar Medical Journal. 2009;**1**:19

[5] Sliwa K, Mebazaa A, Hilifiker-Kleiner D, et al. Clinical characteristics of patients from worldwide registry on peripartum cardiomyopathy (PPCM): EURObservational research program in conjunction with heart failure association of the European society of cardiology study group on PPCM. European Journal of Heart Failure. 2017;**19**:1131

[6] Veille JC. Peripartum cardiomyopathy: A review. American Journal of Obstetrics and Gynecology. 1984;**148**:805

[7] Mendelson MA, Chandler J. Postpartum cardiomyopathy associated with maternal cocaine abuse. The American Journal of Cardiology. 1992;**70**:1092-1094

[8] Lampert MB, Hibbard J, Weinest L, Briller J, Lindheimer M, Lang RM. Peripartum cardiomyopathy associated with prolonged tocolytic therapy. American Journal of Obstetrics and Gynecology. 1993;**168**:493

[9] Hibbard J, Linheumer M, Lany RM. Modified definition for peripartum cardiomyopathy and prognosis based on echocardiography. Obstetrics & Gynecology. 1999;**94**:311

[10] Bello N, Rendon IS, Ricke-Hoch M, et al. The relationship between pre-eclampsia and peripartum cardiomyopathy: A systemic review and met analysis. Journal of the American College of Cardiology. 2013;**62**:1715

[11] Murali S, Baldisseri MR. Peripartum cardiomyopathy. Critical Care Medicine. 2005;**33**:S340

[12] Kao DP, Hsich E, Lindenfeld J. Characteristics, adverse events, and racial differences among delivering mothers with peripartum cardiomyopathy. JACC: Heart Failure. 2013;**1**:409

[13] Melvin KR, Richardson PJ, Olsen EG, Daly K, Jackson G. Peripartum cardiomyopathy due to myocarditis. The New England Journal of Medicine. 1982;**307**:731-734

[14] Pearson GD, Veille JC, Rahimtoola S, Hsia J, Oakley CM, Hosenpud JD, et al. Peripartum cardiomyopathy: National heart lung and blood institute and office of rare disease, workshop recommendations and review. Journal of the American Medical Association. 2000;**283**:1183-1188

[15] Sliwa K, Skudicky D, Bergemann A, et al. Peripartum cardiomyopathy: Analysis of clinical outcome, left ventricular function, plasma levels of cytokines and Fas/APO-1. Journal of the American College of Cardiology. 2000;**35**:701

[16] Cénac A, Beaufils H, Soumana I, et al. Absence of humoral autoimmunity in peripartum cardiomyopathy. A comparative study in Niger. International Journal of Cardiology. 1990;**26**:49

[17] Homans DC. Peripartum cardiomyopathy. The New England Journal of Medicine. 1985;**312**:1432-1437

[18] Patten IS, Rana S, Shahul S, et al. Cardiac angiogenic imbalance leads to peripartum cardiomyopathy. Nature. 2012;**485**:333

[19] Arany Z, Elkayam U. Peripartum cardiomyopathy. Circulation. 2016;**133**:1397-1409

[20] Halkein J, Tabruyn SP, Ricke-Hoch M, et al. MicroRNA-146a is a therapeutic target and biomarker for peripartum cardiomyopathy. The Journal of Clinical Investigation. 2013;**123**:2143

[21] Sliwa K, Förster O, Libhaber E, et al. Peripartum cardiomyopathy: Inflammatory markers as predictors of outcome in 100 prospectively studied patients. European Heart Journal. 2006;**27**:441

[22] Mebazaa A, Seronde MF, Gayat E, et al. Imbalanced angiogenesis in peripartum cardiomyopathy-diagnostic value of placenta growth factor. Circulation Journal. 2017;**81**:1654

[23] Honigberg MC, Givertz MM. Arrhythmias in peripartum cardiomyopathy. Cardiac Electrophysiology Clinics. 2015;**7**:309

[24] Cooper LT, Gersh BJ. Viral infection, inflammation and risk of idiopathic dilated cardiomyopathy. The American Journal of Cardiology. 2002;**90**:751-754

[25] Mouquet F, Mostefa Kara M, Lamblin N, et al. Unexpected and rapid recovery of left ventricular function in patients with peripartum cardiomyopathy: Impact of cardiac resynchronization therapy. European Journal of Heart Failure. 2012;**14**:526

[26] Neumann A, Hilfiker-Kleiner D, Kühn C, et al. Prolactin—A new marker for ECMO-related mortality. The Journal of Heart and Lung Transplantation. 2013;**32**:S225

[27] Loyaga-Rendon RY, Pamboukian SV, Tallaj JA, et al. Outcomes of patients with peripartum cardiomyopathy who received mechanical circulatory support. Data from the interagency registry for mechanically assisted circulatory support. Circulation Heart Failure. 2014;**7**:300

[28] Rasmusson K, Brunisholz K, Budge D, et al. Peripartum cardiomyopathy: Post-transplant outcomes from the united network for organ sharing database. The Journal of Heart and Lung Transplantation. 2012;**31**:180

[29] Sliwa K, Blauwet L, Tibazarwa K, et al. Evaluation of bromocriptine in the treatment of acute severe peripartum cardiomyopathy: A proof-of-concept pilot study. Circulation. 2010;**121**:1465

[30] Hilfiker-Kleiner D, Haghikia A, Berliner D, et al. Bromocriptine for the treatment of peripartum cardiomyopathy: A multicentre randomized study. European Heart Journal. 2017;**38**:2671

[31] Mason JW, O'Connell JB, Herskowitz A, et al. A clinical trial of immunosuppressive therapy for myocarditis. The myocarditis treatment trial investigators. The New England Journal of Medicine. 1995;**333**:269

[32] Safirstein JG, Ro AS, Grandhi S, et al. Predictors of left ventricular recovery in a cohort of peripartum cardiomyopathy patients recruited via the internet. International Journal of Cardiology. 2012;**154**:27

[33] Lee W, Cotton DB. Cardiomyopathy: Current concept and clinical management. Clinical Obstetrics and Gynecology. 1989;**32**:54-67

[34] Felker CM, Thompson RE, Hare JM, et al. The New England Journal of Medicine. 2000;**342**:1077

[35] Harper MA, Meyer RE, Berg CJ. Peripartum cardiomyopathy: Population-based birth prevalence and 7-year mortality. Obstetrics and Gynecology. 2012;**120**:1013

[36] Goland S, Modi K, Bitar F, et al. Clinical profile and predictors of complications in peripartum cardiomyopathy. Journal of Cardiac Failure. 2009;**15**:645

[37] Elkayam U, Akhter MW, Singh H, et al. Pregnancy-associated cardiomyopathy: Clinical characteristics and a comparison between early and late presentation. Circulation. 2005;**111**:2050

[38] Tepper NK, Paulen ME, Marchbanks PA, Curtis KM. Safety of contraceptive use among women with peripartum cardiomyopathy: A systematic review. Contraception. 2010;**82**:95

Chapter 9

Application of Medical Imaging in Diagnosis and Assessment of Myocarditis and Pericarditis

Yousif Mohamed Y. Abdallah and Nouf H. Abuhadi

Abstract

Medical imaging is of one of the most essential means in the investigation of cardiac disorders. In patients, the detection of the whole heart and its adjacent tissues is a crucial procedure since it helps in myocarditis and pericarditis managements. Weekly, there are millions of cardiac imaging performed globally. Medical imaging and processing techniques such as image segmentation, augmentation, and scrutiny can detect cardiac lesions rapidly and precisely. This chapter discusses the application of medical imaging in the diagnosis of myocarditis and pericarditis. This chapter also summarized how to demonstrate image interpretation challenges using diverse image processing procedures and techniques.

Keywords: medical imaging, diagnosis, myocarditis, pericarditis

1. Introduction

The pericardium is a muscular sac that covers the heart and cases its major blood vessels. It facilitates and greases the heart motions [1–3]. In embryonic stage, the internal layer of the pericardium forms the myocardium prior fused with the exterior layer of the fibrous layer [4–7]. Those layers are a few millimeters thick and they are separated from each other. The pericardium gets the blood from inner mammary arteries and its inversion from the phrenic nerve [8, 9]. The pericardium separates from the sternum, vertebral bodies, and diaphragm through many ligaments (**Figure 1**) [10].

The symptoms of myocarditis are common especially in middle-aged patients [11]. Those diseases can cause discomfort, chest pain, tiredness, breathlessness, and repeated visits to clinics. The coronary vessel disease is one of the causes of myocarditis and pericarditis [12–14]. The virus infection is the main cause of myocarditis. This infection is usually associated with serve viral infection. This infection may cause the injury to the myocardium tissues, and it is associated with the accumulation of fluid and local death of tissue, contingent on its nature and extent [15–18]. Fungal infections are infrequent and include aspergillosis, blastomycosis, and candidasis. The tissue can be recovered within days. In acute cases, complete functional tissues work within weeks [19]. Cardiomyopathy may cause the consequences of the chronic inflammatory process (**Figure 2**) [20, 21].

The causes of occurrence of acute myocarditis are idiopathic. Pericarditis is an inflammatory process that affects the pericardium tissues. The signs of pericarditis

IntechOpen

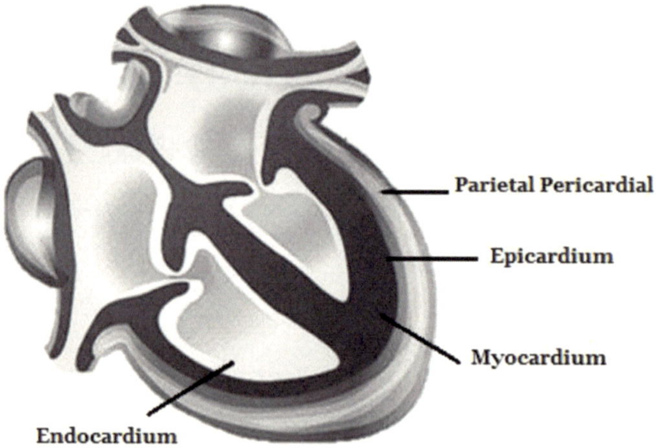

Figure 1.
Shows the pericardium layers.

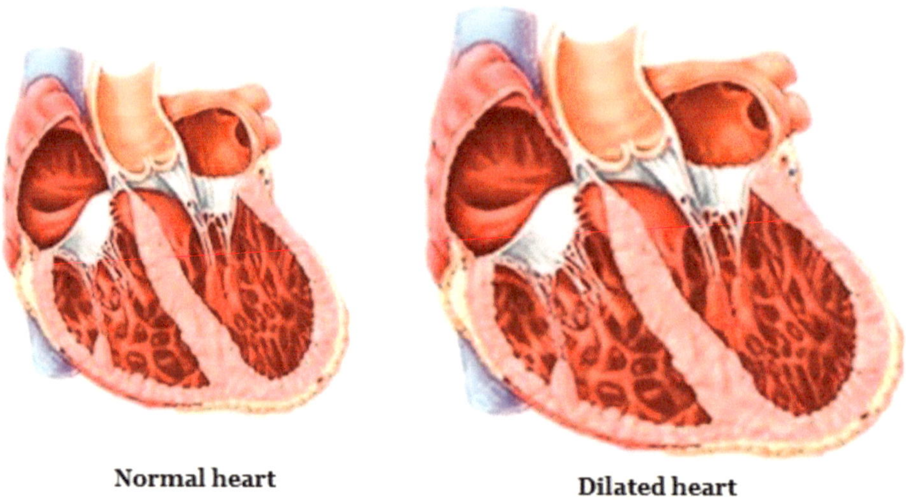

Figure 2.
Shows dilated heart.

are rub, abnormal ECG findings and possible pericardial effusion, chest discomfort, and breathing difficulties. The pericardial rub is best heard at the end of the expiration phase with patient sloping frontward [22–24]. About 30% of patients with myocarditis might be accompanied with pericarditis. Pericarditis is difficult to detect. Some postmortem studies suggest that pericarditis is a subclinical type. Pericarditis accounts for 5% of patients who are attending to emergency rooms due to myocardial infraction and chest discomfort [25–29]. On laboratory results, pericarditis can be detected in a troponin I test. Nevertheless, the elevation of troponin (I) is not used as the adverse prognosis of the disease [30, 31]. Serology may approve the cause as infectious or autoimmune pericarditis. Acute pericarditis onsets with mild signs and symptoms and its treatment lasts for 6 weeks. The infection symptoms might reoccur within 4–6 weeks [32, 33]. The prevalence of pericarditis may include idiopathic, tuberculosis, viral (HIV infection) or systemic infection, cancer (breast, leukemia, lymphoma, and lung), radiation therapy (about 4% of mediastinal Hodgkin's disease), cardiac surgery (20% of the cases of bypass graft surgery), and percutaneous heart examinations [34–36]. The bacterium spreads to the pericardium by blood or direct extension of the adjacent organs. Incidence of myocarditis has been stated after smallpox immunization. The neoplastic pericardium is a secondary cause of the pericarditis [37]. Patients with acute pericarditis have progressive disease and discomfort. This discomfort gets worse when the patient is lying supine. The pain in the area refers to the trapezius muscles and phrenic nerve. Fever might accompany the viral pericarditis [38–40]. Electrocardiogram (ECG) is the most frequent tool for acute pericarditis study. It shows a saddle shape that reflects subepicardium infection. In ECG graph, acute pericarditis shows no Q-wave and loss of R-wave. Imaging of the cardiac tissue has a limited role especially in uncomplicated acute pericarditis. Chest radiographs show the cardiomegaly and pericardial effusion (250 mL). Ultrasound imaging (M-mode and Doppler) is used to differentiate constrictive and restrictive cardiomyopathy. In the pediatric, a transesophageal probe is used to detect diastolic dysfunction. Cytological examinations of pericarditis include glucose, protein, cell count, bacteria and virus culture, and gram and Ziehl-Neelsen stain test. Myolemma and sarcolemma can detect immune-mediated pericarditis. In neoplastic conditions, the high level of the carcinoembryonic antigen is detected. Pericardial biopsy is performed in the granulomatous or malignant suspicion [41–43].

2. Clinical presentation of myocarditis and pericarditis

The medical signs of acute pericarditis and myocarditis include malaise, rash, tiredness, arthralgias, and respiratory and digestive syndromes. The acute infection continues for few weeks. Patients might attend the clinic with chest discomfort, breathlessness, tiredness, and syncope. Cardiac beat disorders are common and include both atrial and ventricular with the possibility of atrioventricular blockage. The European study of the inflammatory disease showed that 72% had dyspnea and 32% chest discomfort. The medical signs in pediatric patients differ according to their age. Kids may have anxiety, tiredness, raised temperature, loss of appetite, increased breath rate, increased heartbeats, and blue skin due to lack of oxygen. Symptoms in toddlers might comprise of chest and abdominal discom fort, muscle pain, tiredness, cough, and fluid accumulation in tissues. The degree of symptoms is reliant on the age of the kid. Toddlers often have and might require progressive cardiovascular and respiratory care in the initial phases of their disease than adults [44].

3. Medical imaging in diagnosis and assessment of myocarditis and pericarditis

3.1 Electrocardiography

Echocardiography is beneficial for assessing cardiac tissue dimensions, wall width, systolic and diastolic, and intracavitary thrombi. This technique can assess cardiac failure. Myocarditis has no special radiographic features in this technique. Nevertheless, myocarditis is characterized by widened, enlarged, and ischemic cardiomyopathies. This technique is commonly used as a diagnostic tool. The accuracy of electrocardiography for pericarditis and myocarditis is about 47% because ECG findings are basic T-wave deviations (**Figure 3**) [45].

The classical ECG examination is comprised of four stages of changes and it is described in about 50% of cases.

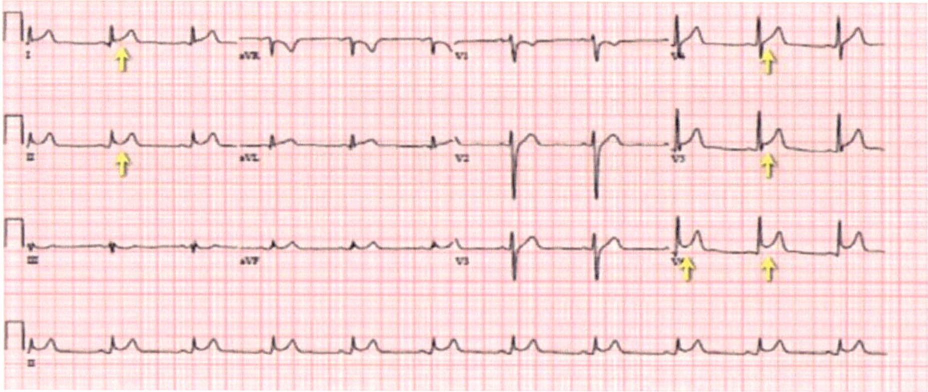

Figure 3.
Shows the ECG scan of myocarditis and pericarditis.

Those stages are:

Stage 1: (hours to a few days): the ST elevation and depression of the PR segment.

Stage 2: (first week): control of the ST and PR segments.

Stage 3: T-wave inversions.

Stage 4: standardization of ECG [46, 47].

3.2 Chest X-ray

Chest radiograph is a radiographic procedure that uses low-energy ionizing radiation (X-rays) to visualize the chest organs. This procedure is very crucial in the assessment of lung and heart signs and symptoms such as cough, chest infection, injury, and discomfort [48]. This procedure is used to evaluate and screen heart inflammatory diseases such as myocarditis and pericarditis. This procedure is noninvasive and does not require special patient preparation. Chest radiography is a standard procedure for myocarditis and pericarditis patients. A distended cardiac shadow might be identified with accumulated fluids. Chest X-ray shows cardiac enlargement as a result of chamber dilatation, pericardial effusion, interstitial infiltrates, and pleural effusions (**Figure 4**) [49–51].

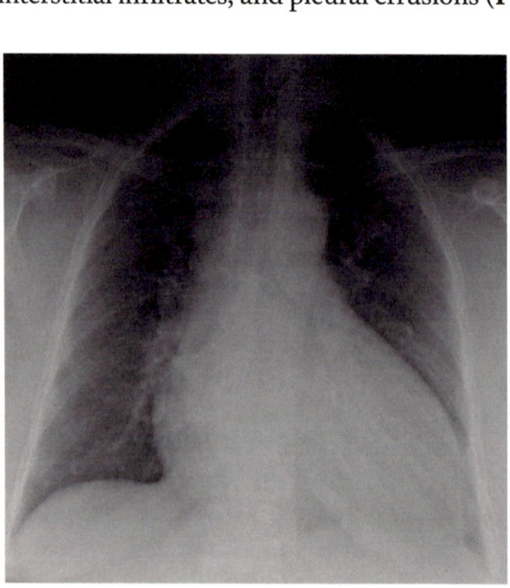

Figure 4.
Shows chest radiograph of myocarditis patient.

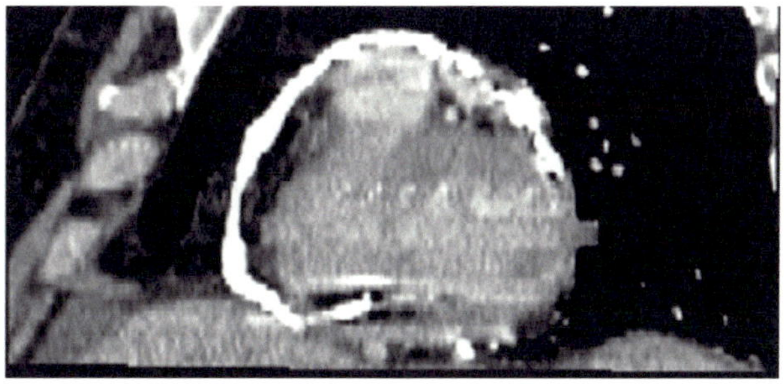

Figure 5.
Shows computed tomography of the pericardium.

3.3 Computed tomography (CT)

Computed tomography provides clear images of pericardium space and infection complications. Nuclear cardiology can delimit the pericarditis. Pericardiocentesis is indicated for pericardial effusion, pus-filled pericarditis, and suspected tumor (**Figure 5**) [52].

3.4 Nuclear medicine

FDG PET-CT can be used for visualization of myocarditis and pericarditis. This technique helps to differentiate between the acute and chronic cardiomyopathy diseases. Recently PET/MRI is used for detecting myocarditis and pericarditis [53]. The evaluation of myocarditis using nuclear scanning had started in the early 1970s. This scanning technique had started by using gallium-67 to visualize the internal

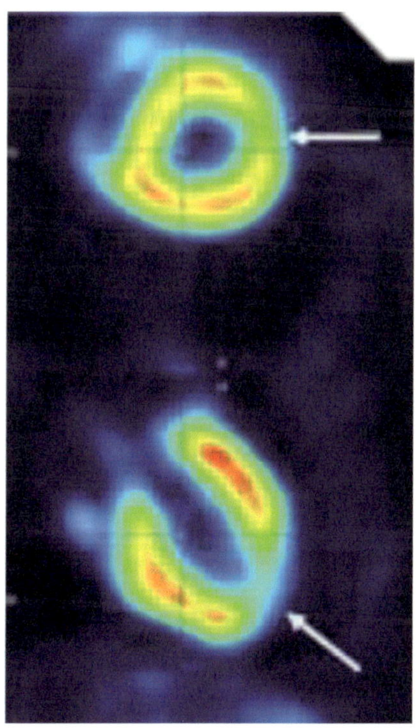

Figure 6.
Shows the nuclear medicine image of myocarditis.

muscles of the heart. In the early 1980s, the utilization of SPECT enhanced the results of detection of the myocardial tissues. So the detection of the myocarditis and pericarditis became easier than using planar scanner. The radioiodine-labeled (I-111) was introduced in the 1970s. This radioactive test was used to detect monoclonal antimyosin antibodies because of its ability to detect the necrotic area (**Figure 6**) [54].

4. Using cardiovascular magnetic resonance (CMR) in the assessment of myocarditis and pericarditis

Recently, CMR has become a crucial tool for acute myocardial tissue damage. In Europe, CMR represents the differential diagnosis of 1/3 of the cardiac cases [55]. CMR is used to detect the features of myocarditis edema and is related with pericardial fluids, which might be visualized together in images. CMR enables the evaluation of myocardial fluid accumulation and infection process. The CMR gives high accuracy and recognition of the acute inflammatory process, regardless of image quality differences due to the scanner and applied procedure [56, 57]. CMR might detect the accumulation of fluids which represents [58]. The body coil might help in the reduction of acquiesced signal noise, signal scattering, flow suppression, suitable slice width, and sufficient scanning time. Sixteen short-axis views are suggested to decrease the artifacts associated with the sluggish transplanar blood stream. In females, the mild edema is scanned using the signal that normalizes to skeletal muscle in similar slice. The gadolinium (Gd) might increase the recognition of the myocarditis edema especially after using contrast media-sensitive sequence and T1-weighted image. The comparison between the signals, prior and throughout the contrast-enhanced scanning, might show the large volume of edema. Consequently, using the adjacent muscle as reference helps in detecting of the edema area [61–63]. Recently, many studies showed that using Lake Louise criteria does not affect the diagnosis, but they increase the possibilities of the false-positive probability rate (**Figure 7**) [59].

Other studies showed that an amplified Gd enhancement ratio of more than 4.0 is related to patient complications and disease prognosis [60]. T2-weighted images might be used to detect myocardial edema, which indicates the presence of myocarditis. This technique had shown high precision and accuracy. The patients'

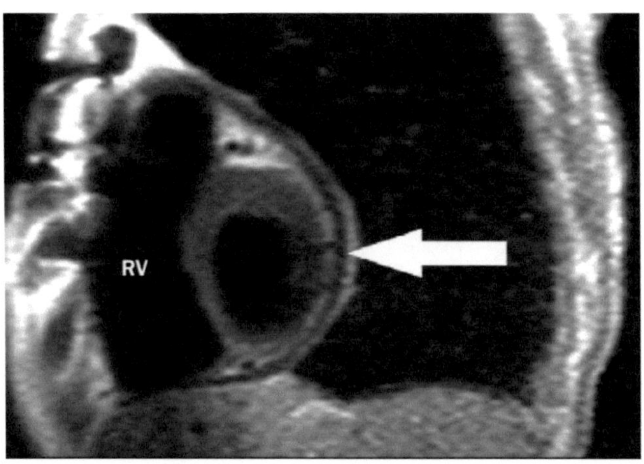

Figure 7.
Shows cardiovascular magnetic resonance of the pericardium.

movements and image artifacts affect the quality of the images. The new scanning protocol overcomes those problems by using the short acquisition time [61–63].

5. Conclusion

Myocardium inflammation is considered as a serious condition that affects both pediatric and adult patients with fetal consequences disease. The chronic myocardial inflammation might eventually lead to cardiac failure. Recently, the evolution in tools of diagnosis, screening, and treatment might decrease the morbidity rate of myocarditis and pericarditis.

About 10% of myocarditis has been discovered in autopsy. Many studies had shown that the best modality to diagnose the myocarditis is a biopsy. Many imaging techniques might be used to diagnose myocarditis and pericarditis; nevertheless, the CMR is the most crucial and precise analytical modality. CMR might help in differentiating between the myocardial infraction, inflammation, and injuries and the degree of severity. The fluoroscopic endomyocardial procedures have low complications compared with other invasive tools. The advance CMR protocols are used to improve the diagnosis and reduce the morbidity.

Acknowledgements

The authors are thankful to the Deanship of Scientific Research, at Majmaah University, for funding this research.

Conflict of interest

There are no conflicts of interest.

Author details

Yousif Mohamed Y. Abdallah[1]* and Nouf H. Abuhadi[2]

1 Radiological Science and Medical Imaging Department, College of Applied Medical Science, Majmaah University, Majmaah, Saudi Arabia

2 Diagnostic Radiology Department, College of Applied Medical Science, Jazan University, Jazan, Saudi Arabia

*Address all correspondence to: y.yousif@mu.edu.sa

IntechOpen

© 2019 The Author(s). Licensee IntechOpen. This chapter is distributed under the terms of the Creative Commons Attribution License (http://creativecommons.org/licenses/by/3.0), which permits unrestricted use, distribution, and reproduction in any medium, provided the original work is properly cited.

References

[1] Assomull RG, Lyne JC, Keenan N, Gulati A, Bunce NH, Davies SW, et al. The role of cardiovascular magnetic resonance in patients presenting with chest pain, raised troponin, and unobstructed coronary arteries. European Heart Journal. 2007;**28**:1242-1249

[2] Cooper LT Jr. Myocarditis. The New England Journal of Medicine. 2009;**360**:1526-1538

[3] Kindermann I, Barth C, Mahfoud F, Ukena C, Lenski M, Yilmaz A, et al. Update on myocarditis. Journal of the American College of Cardiology. 2012;**59**:779-792

[4] Cooper LT, Baughman KL, Feldman AM, Frustaci A, Jessup M, Kuhl U, et al. American Heart Association; American College of Cardiology; European Society of Cardiology. The role of endomyocardial biopsy in the management of cardiovascular disease: A scientific statement from the American Heart Association, the American College of Cardiology, and the European Society of Cardiology. Circulation. 2007;**116**:2216-2233

[5] Jeserich M, Konstantinides S, Pavlik G, Bode C, Geibel A. Non-invasive imaging in the diagnosis of acute viral myocarditis. Clinical Research in Cardiology. 2009;**98**:753-763

[6] Morimoto S, Kato S, Hiramitsu S, Uemura A, Ohtsuki M, Kato Y, et al. Role of myocardial interstitial edema in conduction disturbances in acute myocarditis. Heart and Vessels. 2006;**21**:356-360

[7] Goitein O, Matetzky S, Beinart R, Di Segni E, Hod H, Bentancur A, et al. Acute myocarditis: Noninvasive evaluation with cardiac MRI and transthoracic echocardiography. AJR. American Journal of Roentgenology. 2009;**192**:254-258

[8] Mendes LA, Dec GW, Picard MH, Palacios IF, Newell J, Davidoff R. Right ventricular dysfunction: An independent predictor of adverse outcome in patients with myocarditis. American Heart Journal. 1994;**128**:301-307

[9] Bruder O, Wagner A, Lombardi M, Schwitter J, van Rossum A, Pilz G, et al. European cardiovascular magnetic resonance (EuroCMR) registry–multi national results from 57 centers in 15 countries. Journal of Cardiovascular Magnetic Resonance. 2013;**15**:9

[10] Abdel-Aty H, Boyé P, Zagrosek A, Wassmuth R, Kumar A, Messroghli D, et al. Diagnostic performance of cardiovascular magnetic resonance in patients with suspected acute myocarditis: Comparison of different approaches. Journal of the American College of Cardiology. 2005;**45**:1815-1822

[11] Ong P, Athansiadis A, Hill S, Kispert EM, Borgulya G, Klingel K, et al. Usefulness of pericardial effusion as new diagnostic criterion for noninvasive detection of myocarditis. The American Journal of Cardiology. 2011;**108**:445-452

[12] Grün S, Schumm J, Greulich S, Wagner A, Schneider S, Bruder O, et al. Long-term follow-up of biopsy-proven viral myocarditis: Predictors of mortality and incomplete recovery. Journal of the American College of Cardiology. 2012;**59**:1604-1615

[13] Chu GC, Flewitt JA, Mikami Y, Vermes E, Friedrich MG. Assessment of acute myocarditis by cardiovascular MR: Diagnostic performance of shortened protocols. The International Journal of Cardiovascular Imaging. 2013;**29**:1077-1083

[14] Friedrich MG, Sechtem U, Schulz-Menger J, Holmvang G, Alakija P, Cooper LT, et al. International consensus group on cardiovascular magnetic resonance in myocarditis. Cardiovascular magnetic resonance in myocarditis: A JACC White paper. Journal of the American College of Cardiology. 2009;**53**:1475-1487

[15] American College of Cardiology Foundation Task Force on Expert Consensus Documents, Hundley WG, Bluemke DA, Finn JP, Flamm SD, Fogel MA, et al. ACCF/ACR/AHA/NASCI/SCMR 2010 Expert Consensus Document on Cardiovascular Magnetic Resonance: A Report of the American College of Cardiology Foundation Task Force on Expert Consensus Documents. Vol. 552010. pp. 2614-2662

[16] Friedrich MG, Larose E, Patton D, Dick A, Merchant N, Paterson I. Canadian society for CMR. Canadian Society for Cardiovascular Magnetic Resonance (CanSCMR) recommendations for cardiovascular magnetic resonance image analysis and reporting. The Canadian Journal of Cardiology. 2013;**29**:260-265

[17] Zagrosek A, Wassmuth R, Abdel-Aty H, Rudolph A, Dietz R, Schulz-Menger J. Relation between myocardial edema and myocardial mass during the acute and convalescent phase of myocarditis—A CMR study. Journal of Cardiovascular Magnetic Resonance. 2008;**10**:19

[18] Ferreira VM, Piechnik SK, Dall'Armellina E, Karamitsos TD, Francis S, Moore JM, Ntusi N, Holloway C Choudhury RP, Kardos A, Robson MD, Friedrich MG*, Neubauer S. T1-mapping for the Diagnosis of Acute Myocarditis Using Cardiovascular Magnetic Resonance: Comparison to T2-weighted and Late Gadolinium Enhancement. JACC: Cardiovascular Imaging. 2013;**6**(10):1048-1058

[19] Eitel I, von Knobelsdorff-Brenkenhoff F, Bernhardt P, Carbone I, Muellerleile K, Aldrovandi A, et al. Clinical characteristics and cardiovascular magnetic resonance findings in stress (takotsubo) cardiomyopathy. JAMA. 2011;**306**:277-286

[20] Dall'Armellina E, Piechnik SK, Ferreira VM, Si QL, Robson MD, Francis JM, et al. Cardiovascular magnetic resonance by non contrast T1-mapping allows assessment of severity of injury in acute myocardial infarction. Journal of Cardiovascular Magnetic Resonance. 2012;**14**:15

[21] O h-Ici D, Ridgway JP, Kuehne T, Berger F, Plein S, Sivananthan M, et al. Cardiovascular magnetic resonance of myocardial edema using a short inversion time inversion recovery (STIR) black-blood technique: Diagnostic accuracy of visual and semi-quantitative assessment. Journal of Cardiovascular Magnetic Resonance. 2012;**14**:22

[22] Monney PA, Sekhri N, Burchell T, Knight C, Davies C, Deaner A, et al. Acute myocarditis presenting as acute coronary syndrome: Role of early cardiac magnetic resonance in its diagnosis. Heart. 2011;**97**:1312-1318

[23] Ferreira VM, Piechnik SK, Dall'Armellina E, Karamitsos TD, Francis JM, Choudhury RP, et al. Noncontrast T1-mapping detects acute myocardial edema with high diagnostic accuracy: A comparison to T2-weighted cardiovascular magnetic resonance. Journal of Cardiovascular Magnetic Resonance. 2012;**14**:42

[24] Cocker MS, Abdel-Aty H, Strohm O, Friedrich MG. Age and gender effects on the extent of myocardial involvement in acute myocarditis: A cardiovascular magnetic resonance study. Heart. 2009;**95**:1925-1930

[25] Jerosch-Herold M, Sheridan DC, Kushner JD, Nauman D, Burgess D,

Dutton D, et al. Cardiac magnetic resonance imaging of myocardial contrast uptake and blood flow in patients affected with idiopathic or familial dilated cardiomyopathy. American Journal of Physiology. Heart and Circulatory Physiology. 2008;**295**:H1234-H1242

[26] Wagner A, Schulz-Menger J, Dietz R, Friedrich MG. Long-term followup of patients paragraph sign with acute myocarditis by magnetic paragraph sign resonance imaging. Magma. 2003;**16**:17-20

[27] Mavrogeni S, Spargias C, Bratis C, Kolovou G, Markussis V, Papadopoulou E, et al. Myocarditis as a precipitating factor for heart failure: Evaluation and 1-year follow-up using cardiovascular magnetic resonance and endomyocardial biopsy. European Journal of Heart Failure. 2011;**13**:830-837

[28] Eitel I, Kubusch K, Strohm O, Desch S, Mikami Y, de Waha S, et al. Prognostic value and determinants of a hypointense infarct core in T2-weighted cardiac magnetic resonance in acute reperfused ST infarction. Circulation. Cardiovascular Imaging. 2011;**4**:354-362

[29] Kabbani SS, LeWinter MM. Pericardial diseases. Current Treatment Options in Cardiovascular Medicine. 2002;**4**:487-495

[30] Spodick DH. Colchicine effectively and safely treats acute pericarditis and prevents and treats recurrent pericarditides. Heart. 2012;**98**:1035-1036

[31] Spodick DH. Risk prediction in pericarditis: Who to keep in hospital? Heart. 2008;**94**:398-399

[32] Lilly LS. Treatment of acute and recurrent idiopathic pericarditis. Circulation. 2013;**127**:1723-1726

[33] Imazio M. Contemporary management of pericardial diseases. Current Opinion in Cardiology. 2012;**27**:308-317

[34] Imazio M. Pericardial involvement in systemic inflammatory diseases. Heart. 2011;**97**:1882-1892

[35] Imazio M, Brucato A, Barbieri A. Good prognosis for pericarditis with and without myocardial involvement: Results from a multicenter, prospective cohort study. Circulation. 2013;**128**:42-49

[36] Imazio M, Cooper LT. Management of myopericarditis. Expert Review of Cardiovascular Therapy. 2013;**11**:193-201

[37] Soler-Soler J, Sagristà-Sauleda J, Permanyer-Miralda G. Relapsing pericarditis. Heart. 2004;**90**:1364-1368

[38] Imazio M, Brucato A, Cemin R, et al. ICAP investigators. A randomized trial of colchicine for acute pericarditis. The New England Journal of Medicine. 2013;**369**:1522-1528

[39] Hoit BD. Management of effusive and constrictive pericardial heart disease. Circulation. 2002;**105**:2939-2942

[40] Sagristà-Sauleda J, Angel J, Sánchez A, et al. Effusive-constrictive pericarditis. The New England Journal of Medicine. 2004;**350**:469-475

[41] Imazio M, Cecchi E, Demichelis B, et al. Myopericarditis versus viral or idiopathic acute pericarditis. Heart. 2008;**94**:498-501

[42] Syed FF, Ntsekhe M, Gumedze F, et al. Myopericarditis in tuberculous pericardial effusion: Prevalence, predictors and outcome. Heart. 2014;**100**:135-139

[43] Ntsekhe M, Mayosi BM. Tuberculous pericarditis with and without HIV. Heart Failure Reviews. 2013;**18**:367-373

[44] Permanyer-Miralda G. Acute pericardial disease: Approach to the aetiologic diagnosis. Heart. 2004;**90**:252-254

[45] Snyder MJ, Bepko J, White M. Acute pericarditis: diagnosis and management. American Family Physician. 2014;**89**:553-560

[46] Rossello X, Wiegerinck RF, Alguersuari J. New electrocardiographic criteria to differentiate acute pericarditis and myocardial infarction. The American Journal of Medicine. 2014;**127**:233-239

[47] Klein AL, Abbara S, Agler DA, et al. American Society of Echocardiography clinical recommendations for multimodality cardiovascular imaging of patients with pericardial disease: Endorsed by the Society for Cardiovascular Magnetic Resonance and Society of cardiovascular computed tomography. Journal of the American Society of Echocardiography. 2013;**26**:9651012

[48] Rigante D, Cantarini L, Imazio M, et al. Autoinflammatory diseases and cardiovascular manifestations. Annals of Medicine. 2011;**43**:341-346

[49] Cantarini L, Rigante D, Merlini G, et al. The expanding spectrum of low-penetrance TNFRSF1A gene variants in adults presenting with recurrent inflammatory attacks: Clinical manifestations and long-term follow-up. Seminars in Arthritis and Rheumatism. 2014;**43**:818-823

[50] Abu Fanne R, Banai S, Chorin U, et al. Diagnostic yield of extensive infectious panel testing in acute pericarditis. Cardiology. 2011;**119**:134-139

[51] Lazaros G, Vlachopoulos C, Stefanadis C. Extensive infectious panel testing for acute pericarditis: A ghost hunt? Cardiology. 2011;**119**:131-133

[52] Sagristá Sauleda J, Almenar Bonet L, Angel Ferrer J, et al. The clinical practice guidelines of the Sociedad Española de Cardiología on pericardial pathology. Revista Española de Cardiología. 2000;**53**:394-412

[53] Yared K, Baggish AL, Picard MH, et al. Multimodality imaging of pericardial diseases. JACC: Cardiovascular Imaging. 2010;**3**:650-660

[54] Verhaert D, Gabriel RS, Johnston D, et al. The role of multimodality imaging in the management of pericardial disease. Circulation. Cardiovascular Imaging. 2010;**3**:333-343

[55] Horneffer PJ, Miller RH, Pearson TA, et al. The effective treatment of postpericardiotomy syndrome after cardiac operations. A randomized placebo-controlled trial. The Journal of Thoracic and Cardiovascular Surgery. 1990;**100**:292-296

[56] Lotrionte M, Biondi-Zoccai G, Imazio M, et al. International collaborative systematic review of controlled clinical trials on pharmacologic treatments for acute pericarditis and its recurrences. American Heart Journal. 2010;**160**:662-670

[57] Vianello F, Cinetto F, Cavraro M, et al. Azathioprine in isolated recurrent pericarditis: A single Centre experience. International Journal of Cardiology. 2011;**147**:477-478

[58] Abdallah Y. Improvement of sonographic appearance using HAT-TOP methods. International Journal of Science and Research (IJSR). 2015;**4**(2):2425-2430

[59] Abdallah Y. Increasing of edges recognition in cardiac Scintigraphy for ischemic patients. Journal of Biomedical Engineering and Medical Imaging. 2016;**2**(6):39-40

[60] Abdallah Y. Increasing of Edges Recognition in Cardiac Scintography for Ischemic Patients. Berlin, Germany: Lambert Publishing Press GmbH & Co. KG; 2011. pp. 123-125

[61] Abdallah YM. History of medical imaging. Archives of Medicine and Health Sciences. 2017;**5**:275-278

[62] Abdallah Y. An Introduction to PACS in Radiology Service: Theory and Practice. Vol. 2. Berlin, Germany: LAP LAMBERT Academic Publishing; 2012. pp. 140-153

[63] Abdallah Y, Wagiallah E, Yousef M. Improvement of nuclear cardiology images for ischemic patients using image processing techniques. SMU Medical Journal. 2015;**2**(2):2415-2419

Section 3

Atherosclerotic Cardiovascular Disease

Chapter 10

Atherosclerosis at Extracranial Carotid Vessels and Serum Homocysteine

Mei-Ling Sharon Tai, Kuo Ghee Ong, Tsun Haw Toh, Hafez Hussain, Abdul Rashid Mat Mahidin and Esther Kar Mun Yeow

Abstract

In this chapter we will discuss more about the role of homocysteine in atherosclerosis and also association between serum homocysteine with extracranial carotid atherosclerosis. Carotid atherosclerosis comprises an increase in carotid intima-media (CIMT) thickening, plaque formation and carotid stenosis. Atherogenic property of homocysteine was discovered in 1969. Atherosclerosis is initiated by endothelial dysfunction. One of the causes of endothelial abnormality is homocysteine. The development of aggregates of homocysteinylated lipoproteins with microorganisms obstructs the vasa vasorum in vulnerable plaques. In one study, serum homocysteine in the highest quartile was independently associated with extracranial carotid artery stenosis ≥50%. In another study, raised serum homocysteine was also independently associated with severe extracranial carotid stenosis in both genders. In other studies, serum homocysteine was significantly associated with carotid artery stenosis in internal carotid arteries and external carotid arteries as well as the degree of stenosis. The hypertensive patients who had raised serum homocysteine were reported to have higher risk of developing asymptomatic extracranial carotid artery stenosis.

Keywords: homocysteine, carotid, extracranial, atherosclerosis, stenosis

1. History

Premature atherosclerosis was first reported by McCully in 1969 [1]. He described it on two infant patients with raised homocysteine with similar arterial changes [1]. These two patients had large- and medium-sized arterial narrowing [1]. The histology was focal fibrosis of intima and media layers, focal proliferation of perivascular connective tissue of small arteries, as well as prominent internal elastic membranes in medium- and small-sized arteries [1].

Since then, numerous studies on homocysteine have been conducted. The level of homocysteine-cysteine mixed disulphide after a methionine load was shown to be slightly higher in the patients with coronary artery disease (CAD) in 1976 [2]. In addition, the fasting level of serum homocysteine was 31% higher in the patients with all vascular diseases than in controls [3]. Raised serum homocysteine was found to be an independent risk factor for vascular diseases with odds ratios (OR) of 1.5 to 1.8 for every increase of 5 μmol/L in serum homocysteine [4]. In a meta-analysis, raised serum homocysteine was an independent predictor of ischaemic stroke and CAD in the healthy population [5].

2. Introduction: molecular aspects of homocysteine

Homocysteine is a sulphur-containing amino acid which is derived from methionine [6]. Methionine is activated by ATP to S-adenosylmethionine (SAM) [6]. In turn, S-adenosylhomocysteine (SAH) is produced from SAM by transmethylation process [6]. Subsequently, SAH is then hydrolysed into homocysteine [6].

Cystathionine β-synthase (CBS) has the role of catalysing the condensation of homocysteine together with serine into cystathionine by process of transsulfuration [6]. The conversion of cystathionine into cysteine depends on pyridoxal 5′-phosphate [6].

3. Introduction to extracranial carotid atherosclerosis

Cardiovascular diseases due to atherosclerosis include ischaemic stroke, transient ischaemic attack (TIA), CAD and peripheral vascular disease [7]. One of the causes of ischaemic stroke is the atherosclerosis involving the extracranial carotid arteries [8, 9]. Ischaemic stroke occurs secondary to ischemia caused by flow-limiting carotid artery stenosis or by embolism due to plaque rupture [8]. 20–30% of ischaemic strokes in the Western countries are caused by stenosis or occlusion of the extracranial carotid arteries [7].

Atherosclerosis is initiated by endothelial dysfunction [10, 11]. This endothelial abnormality is mainly caused by free radicals, homocysteine, lipoproteins, free radicals and infectious agents [10, 11]. In addition, atherosclerosis develops by activation and proliferation of smooth muscle cells [10, 11]. This leads to thickening of the arterial wall [10, 11]. Moreover, there is infiltration of macrophages which result in fatty streak and plasma-derived extracellular lipid accumulation in the thickened intima layer [10–12].

Beginning in the mid-1980s, subclinical atherosclerosis was assessed by measurement of carotid intima-media thickness with ultrasound carotid Doppler [13]. Later, other parameters such as carotid plaques were used to evaluate for atherosclerosis [14]. These parameters of subclinical atherosclerosis are useful in assessment of cardiovascular diseases, such as CAD and ischaemic stroke [15–18].

The frequency of ipsilateral strokes was higher in the patients with progressive asymptomatic carotid stenosis than those without asymptomatic carotid stenosis [19]. A rate of 5.3% of developing ipsilateral strokes was observed in the patients with moderate asymptomatic carotid stenosis [19].

The presence of extracranial carotid artery stenosis was found to be negatively associated with ideal baseline cardiovascular health in several studies [20, 21]. An assessment of carotid intima-media thickness (CIMT) is a good indicator of coronary atherosclerosis [22, 23]. In addition, CIMT is an independent predictor of cardiovascular mortality [22, 23]. Moreover, reduced frequency of subclinical atherosclerosis is associated with ideal cardiovascular health profile [24]. Several large population studies showed that there was an association between increased CIMT with future cardiovascular events [25]. In the Multi-Ethnic Study of Atherosclerosis (MESA), Zhang et al. reported that measurement of CIMT with magnetic resonance imaging (MRI) was more consistently associated with incident cardiovascular diseases (especially stroke) than ultrasound carotid [26].

The presence of carotid plaque helps in the identification of the patients with coronary atherosclerosis [14]. The baseline plaque area is believed to be more than 3.4 times more powerful than the Framingham risk Equation [27]. The patients with plaque scores in the highest quartile had 3.4 times higher risk of stroke, myocardial infarction and overall mortality in the last 5 years than those in the lowest quartile [27]. Measurement of plaque area is a sensitive parameter to assess atherosclerosis [28]. In a recent study by Kaspar et al., ultrasound-based carotid plaque analysis techniques are more promising for future research studies on generalised atherosclerosis [25].

4. Pathophysiology

Raised serum homocysteine results in endothelial dysfunction as manifested by changes in endothelial cell structure and function [29, 30]. The hypothesised mechanisms were pro-inflammatory effects (expression of tumour necrosis factor-α and inducible nitric oxide (NO) synthase), oxidative stress and impaired endothelium-mediated platelet inhibition [31–33]. In addition, raised serum homocysteine leads to a decrease in nitric oxide bioavailability and inflammation [30].

The autoxidation of homocysteine produces oxidative stress [32]. Raised serum homocysteine-related pathologies such as atherosclerosis and thrombosis are believed to be due to oxidative stress [34–37]. Hydroxyl free radicals due to raised serum homocysteine level remove electrons from other molecules including DNA, proteins, lipids and carbohydrates in all the cellular components [34–37]. In addition, the hydroxyl free radicals stimulate lipid oxidation and accumulate intracellular cholesterol [33]. Raised serum homocysteine level increases the adhesion between the endothelial cells and neutrophils, resulting in release of extracellular hydrogen peroxide which damages the endothelial cell [38].

Homocysteine is important in vascular function and atherosclerosis [39]. Ozone activates thioretinaco to produce thioretinaco ozonide which is the active site for oxidative phosphorylation [40]. In addition, ozone has been discovered to be present in human atherosclerotic plaques, thus emphasising the important role of ozone and cholesterol ozonolysis in atherosclerosis [41]. Aggregates of microorganisms, homocysteinylated and oxidised low-density lipoproteins (LDL) and lipoprotein autoantibodies in regions of high pressure lead to obstruction of the vasa vasorum [39, 42, 43]. This in turn results in ischaemia and rupture into arterial intima to form the vulnerable plaque [39, 42, 43].

Endothelial cell hyperplasia and fibrin deposition in the walls of arterioles may worsen the degree of obstruction of the vasa vasorum by lipoprotein aggregates [1]. Homocysteine activates the proliferation of endothelial cells by inhibiting the nitric oxide production by platelets and endothelial cells [37, 44]. Subsequently, production of glutathione peroxidase is suppressed, and this results in a rise of amount of arachidonic acid from platelets to produce more reactive oxygen species [37].

Homocysteine initiates the coagulation process by tissue factor pathway [45]. Homocysteine activates platelet production of the thromboxane A2, a vasoconstrictor and pro-aggregant [46]. Moreover, homocysteine causes thrombosis by inhibiting tissue plasminogen activator binding domain of annexin II [47]. Homocysteine suppresses the activation of protein C and thrombomodulin surface expression [48] as well as increases the adhesion of platelets [49].

5. Factors affecting serum homocysteine level

Genetic polymorphisms of the metabolic genes, such as methylenetetrahydrofolate reductase (MTHFR), cystathionine-beta-synthase (CBS), DNA methyltransferase (DNMT) and nicotinamide N-methyl-transferase (NNMT), results in increased level of homocysteine [50, 51]. This leads to an increased risk of ischaemic stroke [50, 51]. CBS deficiency is the most common cause of homocysteinemia due to genetic cause [52]. In the mutation in the gene coding for the enzyme MTHFR, cytosine is replaced by thymidine (C → T) at the base position 677 of the gene [53]. The carriers have nearly 70% reduction in the enzymatic activity [53]. Therefore, the carriers have 20% increase of serum homocysteine concentrations [54]. Deficiencies in CBS and MTHFR result in very high serum homocysteine levels [55].

Nutritional and metabolic abnormalities can also result in elevated serum homocysteine [42]. Metabolism of homocysteine involves remethylation to methionine requiring folate and vitamin B12-derived methylcobalamin [56]. Furthermore, in the process of transsulfuration to cystathionine, vitamin B6-derived pyridoxal 5′-phosphate is needed [56]. Nutritional deficiencies in the vitamin B cofactors inhibit the metabolism of homocysteine metabolism, and this causes an elevated level of serum homocysteine [56].

Serum homocysteine level was significantly higher in the patients with people with impaired renal function [57]. In various studies, gender was significantly correlated with serum homocysteine [53, 58]. However, in some other studies, there was no variation in gender [59].

Parkinsonism and antiepileptic medications have been reported to lead to raised serum homocysteine [60–63]. Paradoxically, lipid-lowering medications have also been reported to cause raised serum homocysteine [60, 63]. The patients with diabetes mellitus (DM) have higher homocysteine than nondiabetics irrespective of gender and ethnic group [64, 65]. Malignancy also leads to higher concentration of homocysteine [66].

6. Factors affecting extracranial carotid atherosclerosis

Atherosclerosis involves inflammation, intimal injury, proliferation of smooth muscle cells and lipid metabolism [67, 68]. In the Framingham study, fasting cholesterol level, systolic blood pressure (SBP), age and status of smoking were significantly associated with the degree of extracranial carotid stenosis in both genders [69]. In the study by Zhu et al., age was correlated positively with CIMT [70]. Hyperlipidaemia, hypertension, DM and smoking were thought to be associated with endothelial dysfunction [71]. In another study, there was positive correlation between incidence of smoking and hypertension with the severity of presentation of extracranial carotid artery stenosis [72].

In a recent study, CIMT and carotid plaques were associated with hypertension, DM and hyperlipidaemia [73]. Male gender has an increased risk of ischaemic stroke in comparison to female gender for all degrees of carotid stenosis [74, 75]. After the age of 85, female gender had a higher risk of stroke [76]. Carotid plaques present in female gender contain reduced level of pro-inflammatory cytokine and more smooth muscle cell content [77]. Female gonadal hormones provide protective effect by causing favourable lipid profile change and by increasing neuronal viability and cerebral blood flow [78, 79]. Oestrogen protects premenopausal women against atherosclerosis [78, 79].

Various ethnic groups have different associations with vascular risk factors [80]. Therefore, these ethnic groups have varying prothrombotic factors and degrees of plaque rupture [80]. Particularly, South Asians have increased serum homocysteine levels in comparison to Chinese and European patients [80]. Kim et al. reported that serum homocysteine is a predictor of asymptomatic carotid stenosis in the patients undergoing coronary artery bypass surgery (CABG) [81].

7. Homocysteine and extracranial carotid artery stenosis

Kim et al. reported that serum homocysteine in the highest quartile was independently associated with extracranial carotid artery stenosis ≥50% [81]. In another study, raised serum homocysteine was also independently associated with severe extracranial carotid stenosis in both genders [82]. In other studies, serum homocysteine was significantly associated with carotid artery stenosis in internal carotid arteries and external carotid arteries as well as the degree of stenosis [83, 84]. The hypertensive patients who had raised serum homocysteine were reported to have higher risk of developing asymptomatic extracranial carotid artery stenosis [85]. However, other studies showed conflicting results [86–87].

In a community-based study, serum homocysteine >19.3 μmol/L was associated with asymptomatic carotid artery stenosis in the non-smoker participants aged ≥40 without transient ischemic attack and coronary artery disease [21]. In addition, raised serum homocysteine was associated with asymptomatic carotid artery stenosis in the diabetic patients [21]. Wang et al. reported that serum homocysteine level of ≥15 μmol/L was a predictor of extracranial carotid stenosis [20] and serum homocysteine level > 14.4 μmol/L was associated with increased extracranial carotid stenosis ≥25% in the elderly people [88], whereas Samson et al. reported that serum homocysteine >10 μmol/L was associated with carotid artery stenosis [89].

Every 1 μmol/L increase of total homocysteine level was associated with 1.12 times the risk for developing internal carotid artery (ICA) occlusion after adjustment for stroke subtypes and risk factors [90]. In the study conducted by Wang et al., every 1 μmol/L increase of total homocysteine level was associated with 1.096 times the risk of developing extracranial carotid stenosis [20]. In addition, Mueller et al. identified serum homocysteine as independent predictor of ICA stenosis ≥50%, with OR 1.32 (95% CI: 1.02–1.72) for every rise of 5 μmol/L [91].

In a previous study, elevated serum homocysteine level is associated with a higher prevalence of 40–100% extracranial carotid arterial disease (ECAD) in older patients [92]. In this study, high serum homocysteine levels were seen in 45% of the older male patients with 40–100% ECAD, whereas only in 20% of the older men with 0–39% ECAD [92]. In addition, elevated serum homocysteine levels were found in 40% of the older female patients with 40–100% ECAD versus 18% of the older women with 0–39% ECAD [92].

Elevated serum homocysteine levels were also associated with a higher prevalence of coronary artery disease (CAD) and peripheral artery disease in older patients [93, 94]. In another study, the significant independent predictors of new cerebral infarction in older patients were serum homocysteine, age, smoking, diabetes mellitus, hypertension and previous cerebral infarcts [95].

Moreover, in a previous study, the significant independent predictors of new-onset CAD in older patients were serum homocysteine, age, smoking, diabetes mellitus, hypertension and hyperlipidaemia [96].

8. Homocysteine and carotid plaque

Increased serum homocysteine level was associated with 1.344 higher risk of developing carotid plaque [97]. Plaque area was reported to be increased in the patients with raised serum homocysteine level [98, 99]. Furthermore, the presence of complicated atheromatous plaque was significantly associated with serum homocysteine level [98].

The patients with serum homocysteine level > 15 μmol/L had increased risk of presence of carotid plaque and plaque in bilateral common carotid artery (CCA) [100]. An increase in serum homocysteine was independently associated with plaque morphology and larger plaque area [101].

The patients with serum homocysteine level of ≥8.6 μmol/L had higher risk of developing echolucent plaques [101]. In another study, the patients with raised serum homocysteine level had 1.28 times risk of developing advanced carotid plaques after adjustment for age and gender [102]. Advanced carotid plaques were defined as ulcerated plaque and plaques with incomplete fibrous cap [102]. These advanced carotid plaques resulted in a higher ischaemic stroke risk [102]. In the study by Zhang et al., raised serum homocysteine acted synergistically with hypertension; therefore there was a greater risk of having plaque in bilateral CCA [100]. Alvarez et al. reported that in the patients with carotid stenosis of more than 70% and were receiving surgical management, high homocysteine level was present in the patients with extracranial cerebrovascular diseases [103].

9. Homocysteine and carotid intima-media thickness

An increase in homocysteine level was significantly associated with an increase in CIMT carotid intima-media thickness [104]. In a study on the patients with primary hypertension, serum homocysteine level was independently associated with CIMT [105]. A significant positive correlation between homocysteine and intima-media thickness was reported [106]. In another study conducted among the patients with Parkinson's disease receiving treatment, there was positive correlation with statistical significance between CIMT and serum homocysteine level [107]. The patients with raised serum homocysteine as well as hypertension had higher risk of increased CIMT [100].

10. Association of serum homocysteine with atherosclerosis

According to Wu et al., there was correlation between serum homocysteine level with carotid intima-media thickness and total number of plaques and unstable plaques [84]. He also reported that serum homocysteine level was correlated with stenosis of ICAs and external carotid arteries (ECA) [84]. In a study on middle-aged asymptomatic women, serum homocysteine was significantly associated with atherosclerosis change after adjustment for age, LDL, diastolic blood pressure and body mass index [108].

In conclusion, raised serum homocysteine should be diagnosed early as this can lead to increased CIMT, carotid plaque and extracranial carotid stenosis. Raised serum homocysteine level can be managed with folic acid and vitamin supplementation.

Acknowledgements

We would like to thank Dr. Lattish Rao Threemurthy and Dr. Parathythasan a/l Rajaandra for their help.

Funding

Supported by University of Malaya UMCares grant RU013-2017C.

Author details

Mei-Ling Sharon Tai[1]*, Kuo Ghee Ong[2], Tsun Haw Toh[1], Hafez Hussain[2], Abdul Rashid Mat Mahidin[2] and Esther Kar Mun Yeow[1]

1 Division of Neurology, Department of Medicine, Faculty of Medicine, University Malaya, Kuala Lumpur, Malaysia

2 SOCSO Tun Razak Rehabilitation Centre, Melaka, Malaysia

*Address all correspondence to: sharont1990@gmail.com

IntechOpen

© 2019 The Author(s). Licensee IntechOpen. This chapter is distributed under the terms of the Creative Commons Attribution License (http://creativecommons.org/licenses/by/3.0), which permits unrestricted use, distribution, and reproduction in any medium, provided the original work is properly cited.

References

[1] McCully KS. Vascular pathology of shomocysteinemia: Implications for the pathogenesis of arteriosclerosis. The American Journal of Pathology. 1969;**56**(1):111

[2] Wilcken D, Wilcken B. The pathogenesis of coronary artery disease. A possible role for methionine metabolism. The Journal of Clinical Investigation. 1976;**57**(4):1079-1082

[3] Ueland PM, Refsum H, Brattstrom L. Plasma Homocysteine and Cardiovascular Disease. Atherosclerotic Cardiovascular Disease, Hemostasis, and Endothelial Function. Vol. 183. New York: Marcel Dekker; 1992

[4] Boushey CJ, Beresford SA, Omenn GS, Motulsky AG. A quantitative assessment of plasma homocysteine as a risk factor for vascular disease: Probable benefits of increasing folic acid intakes. Journal of the American Medical Association. 1995;**274**(13):1049-1057

[5] Collaboration HS. Homocysteine and risk of ischemic heart disease and stroke: A meta-analysis. Journal of the American Medical Association. 2002;**288**(16):2015-2022

[6] Durand P, Prost M, Loreau N, Lussier-Cacan S, Blache D. Impaired homocysteine metabolism and atherothrombotic disease. Laboratory Investigation. 2001;**81**(5):645

[7] Edward IB, Barbara AC. The extracranial cerebral vessels. In: Carol MR, Stephanie RW, Charboneau JW, Deborah L, editors. Diagnostic ultrasound. 4th ed ed. Philadelphia: Elsevier; 2010

[8] Griggs RM, Bluth EI. Noninvasive risk assessment for stroke: Special emphasis on carotid atherosclerosis, sex-related differences, and the development of an effective screening strategy. American Journal of Roentgenology. 2011;**196**(2):259-264

[9] Kolominsky-Rabas PL, Weber M, Gefeller O, Neundoerfer B, Heuschmann PU. Epidemiology of ischemic stroke subtypes according to TOAST criteria: Incidence, recurrence, and long-term survival in ischemic stroke subtypes: A population-based study. Stroke. 2001;**32**(12):2735-2740

[10] Qureshi AR, Alvestrand A, Divino-Filho JC, Gutierrez A, Heimbürger O, Lindholm B, et al. Inflammation, malnutrition, and cardiac disease as predictors of mortality in hemodialysis patients. Journal of the American Society of Nephrology. 2002;**13**(Suppl 1):S28-S36

[11] Stolić R, Trajković G, Šubarić-Gorgieva G. Ultrasound diagnostics of atherosclerosis in chronic renal insufficiency. Medicinski Pregled. 2006;**59**(5-6):270-272

[12] Nakagawa K, Nakashima Y. Pathologic intimal thickening in human atherosclerosis is formed by extracellular accumulation of plasma-derived lipids and dispersion of intimal smooth muscle cells. Atherosclerosis. 2018;**274**:235-242

[13] Bond MG, Strickland HL, Wilmoth SK, Safrit A, Phillips R, Szostak L. Interventional clinical trials using noninvasive ultrasound end points: The multicenter isradipine/diuretic atherosclerosis study. The MIDAS Research Group. Journal of Cardiovascular Pharmacology. 1990;**15**:S30-S33

[14] Spence JD. Technology insight: Ultrasound measurement of carotid plaque—Patient management, genetic research, and therapy evaluation. Nature Reviews. Neurology. 2006;**2**(11):611

[15] Aronow W, Ahn C, Schoenfeld M, Gutstein H. Extracranial carotid arterial disease: A prognostic factor for atherothrombotic brain infarction and cerebral transient ischemic attack. New York State Journal of Medicine. 1992;**92**(10):424-425

[16] Blankenhorn D, Selzer RH, Crawford D, Barth JD, Liu C, Liu C, et al. Beneficial effects of colestipol-niacin therapy on the common carotid artery. Two-and four-year reduction of intima-media thickness measured by ultrasound. Circulation. 1993;**88**(1):20-28

[17] Falke P, Stavenow L. Advanced carotid stenosis in TIA and minor stroke as a predictor of coronary heart disease: A 3-year follow-up. International Angiology: A journal of the International Union of Angiology. 1989;**8**(4):175-178

[18] O'leary DH, Polak JF, Kronmal RA, Kittner SJ, Bond MG, Wolfson SK Jr, et al. Distribution and correlates of sonographically detected carotid artery disease in the cardiovascular health study. The CHS Collaborative Research Group. Stroke. 1992,**23**(12):1752-1760

[19] Kakkos SK, Nicolaides AN, Charalambous I, Thomas D, Giannopoulos A, Naylor AR, et al. Predictors and clinical significance of progression or regression of asymptomatic carotid stenosis. Journal of Vascular Surgery. 2014;**59**(4):956-967

[20] Wang J, Shao B, Da Lin XH, Zhang Y, Zhang L, Jiang T, et al. Ideal cardiovascular health metrics associated with reductions in the risk of extracranial carotid artery stenosis: A population-based cohort study. Scientific Reports. 2018;**8**(1):12277

[21] Jia J, Wang A, Wang J, Wu J, Yan X, Zhou Y, et al. Homocysteine and its relationship to asymptomatic carotid stenosis in a Chinese community population. Scientific Reports. 2016;**6**:37361

[22] Stolić R, Trajković G, Perić V, Jovanović A, Šubarić-Gorgieva G. Impact of arteriosclerosis on the functioning of arteriovenous fistula for hemodialysis. Vojnosanitetski Pregled. 2007;**64**(1):13-18

[23] Crouse JR, Goldbourt U, Evans G, Pinsky J, Sharrett AR, Sorlie P, et al. Risk factors and segment-specific carotid arterial enlargement in the atherosclerosis risk in communities (ARIC) cohort. Stroke. 1996;**27**(1):69-75

[24] Kulshreshtha A, Goyal A, Veledar E, McClellan W, Judd S, Eufinger SC, et al. Association between ideal cardiovascular health and carotid intima-media thickness: A twin study. Journal of the American Heart Association. 2014;**3**(1):e000282

[25] Kaspar M, Baumgartner I, Staub D, Drexel H, Thalhammer C. Non-invasive ultrasound-based imaging of atherosclerosis. Vasa. 2019;**48**:126-133

[26] Zhang Y, Guallar E, Malhotra S, Astor BC, Polak JF, Qiao Y, et al. Carotid artery wall thickness and incident cardiovascular events: A comparison between US and MRI in the multi-ethnic study of atherosclerosis (MESA). Radiology. 2018;**289**(3):649-657

[27] Spence JD, Eliasziw M, DiCicco M, Hackam DG, Galil R, Lohmann T. Carotid plaque area: A tool for targeting and evaluating vascular preventive therapy. Stroke. 2002;**33**(12):2916-2922

[28] Barnett PA, Spence JD, Manuck SB, Jennings JR. Psychological stress and the progression of carotid artery disease. Journal of Hypertension. 1997;**15**(1):49-55

[29] McCully KS. Chemical pathology of homocysteine. IV. Excitotoxicity,

oxidative stress, endothelial dysfunction, and inflammation. Annals of Clinical and Laboratory Science. 2009;**39**(3):219-232

[30] Kumar A, Palfrey HA, Pathak R, Kadowitz PJ, Gettys TW, Murthy SN. The metabolism and significance of homocysteine in nutrition and health. Nutrition & Metabolism (London). 2017;**14**(1):78

[31] Faraci FM, Lentz SR. Hyperhomocysteinemia, oxidative stress, and cerebral vascular dysfunction. Stroke. 2004;**35**(2):345-347

[32] Stanger O, Weger M. Interactions of homocysteine, nitric oxide, folate and radicals in the progressively damaged endothelium. Clinical Chemistry and Laboratory Medicine. 2003;**41**(11):1444-1454

[33] Toole JF, Malinow MR, Chambless LE, Spence JD, Pettigrew LC, Howard VJ, et al. Lowering homocysteine in patients with ischemic stroke to prevent recurrent stroke, myocardial infarction, and death: The vitamin intervention for stroke prevention (VISP) randomized controlled trial. Journal of the American Medical Association. 2004;**291**(5):565-575

[34] Dayal S, Arning E, Bottiglieri T, Böger RH, Sigmund CD, Faraci FM, et al. Cerebral vascular dysfunction mediated by superoxide in hyperhomocysteinemic mice. Stroke. 2004;**35**(8):1957-1962

[35] Herrmann W, Obeid R. Homocysteine: A biomarker in neurodegenerative diseases. Clinical Chemistry and Laboratory Medicine. 2011;**49**(3):435-441

[36] Marković AR, Hrnčić D, Macut D, Stanojlović O, Djuric D. Anticonvulsive effect of folic acid in homocysteine thiolactone-induced seizures. Cellular and Molecular Neurobiology. 2011;**31**(8):1221

[37] Petras M, Tatarkova Z, Kovalska M, Mokra D, Dobrota D, Lehotsky J, et al. Hyperhomocysteinemia as a risk factor for the neuronal system disorders. Journal of Physiology and Pharmacology. 2014;**65**(1):15-23

[38] Dudman NP, Temple SE, Guo XW, Fu W, Perry MA. Homocysteine enhances neutrophil-endothelial interactions in both cultured human cells and rats in vivo. Circulation Research. 1999;**84**(4):409-416

[39] McCully KS. Homocysteine metabolism, atherosclerosis, and diseases of aging. Comprehensive Physiology. 2015;**6**(1):471-505

[40] McCully KS. Chemical pathology of homocysteine. II. Carcinogenesis and homocysteine thiolactone metabolism. Annals of Clinical and Laboratory Science. 1994;**24**(1):27-59

[41] Wentworth P, Nieva J, Takeuchi C, Galve R, Wentworth AD, Dilley RB, et al. Evidence for ozone formation in human atherosclerotic arteries. Science. 2003;**302**(5647):1053-1056

[42] McCully KS. Homocysteine and the pathogenesis of atherosclerosis. Expert Review of Clinical Pharmacology. 2015;**8**(2):211-219

[43] Ravnskov U, McCully KS. Vulnerable plaque formation from obstruction of vasa vasorum by homocysteinylated and oxidized lipoprotein aggregates complexed with microbial remnants and LDL autoantibodies. Annals of Clinical and Laboratory Science. 2009;**39**(1):3-16

[44] Stühlinger MC, Tsao PS, Her J-H, Kimoto M, Balint RF, Cooke JP. Homocysteine impairs the nitric oxide synthase pathway: Role of asymmetric dimethylarginine. Circulation. 2001;**104**(21):2569-2575

[45] Fryer RH, Wilson BD, Gubler DB, Fitzgerald LA, Rodgers GM.

Homocysteine, a risk factor for premature vascular disease and thrombosis, induces tissue factor activity in endothelial cells. Arteriosclerosis and Thrombosis: A Journal of Vascular Biology. 1993;**13**(9):1327-1333

[46] Graeber JE, Slott JH, Ulane RE, Schulman JD, Stuart MJ. Effect of homocysteine and homocystine on platelet and vascular arachidonic acid metabolism. Pediatric Research. 1982;**16**:490

[47] Hajjar KA, Mauri L, Jacovina AT, Zhong F, Mirza UA, Padovan JC, et al. Tissue plasminogen activator binding to the annexin II tail domain direct modulation by homocysteine. The Journal of Biological Chemistry. 1998;**273**(16):9987-9993

[48] Lentz S, Sadler JE. Inhibition of thrombomodulin surface expression and protein C activation by the thrombogenic agent homocysteine. The Journal of Clinical Investigation. 1991;**88**(6):1906-1914

[49] Spence JD. Homocysteine-lowering therapy: A role in stroke prevention? The Lancet Neurology. 2007;**6**(9):830-838

[50] Balcerzyk A, Niemiec P, Kopyta I, Emich-Widera E, Pilarska E, Pienczk-Ręcławowicz K, et al. Methylenetetrahydrofolate reductase gene A1298C polymorphism in pediatric stroke—Case–control and family-based study. Journal of Stroke and Cerebrovascular Diseases. 2015;**24**(1):61-65

[51] Hozyasz KK, Mostowska A, Szaflarska-Poplawska A, Lianeri M, Jagodzinski PP. Polymorphic variants of genes involved in homocysteine metabolism in celiac disease. Molecular Biology Reports. 2012;**39**(3):3123-3130

[52] Mudd SH, Skovby F, Levy HL, Pettigrew KD, Wilcken B, Pyeritz RE, et al. The natural history of homocystinuria due to cystathionine β-synthase deficiency. American Journal of Human Genetics. 1985;**37**(1):1

[53] Stanger O, Herrmann W, Pietrzik K, Fowler B, Geisel J, Dierkes J, et al. DACH-LIGA homocystein (German, Austrian and Swiss homocysteine society): Consensus paper on the rational clinical use of homocysteine, folic acid and B-vitamins in cardiovascular and thrombotic diseases: Guidelines and recommendations. Clinical Chemistry and Laboratory Medicine. 2003;**41**(11):1392-1403

[54] Frosst P, Blom H, Milos R, Goyette P, Sheppard CA, Matthews R, et al. A candidate genetic risk factor for vascular disease: A common mutation in methylenetetrahydrofolate reductase. Nature Genetics. 1995;**10**(1):111

[55] Rozen R. Genetic predisposition to hyperhomocysteinemia: Deficiency of methylenetetrahydrofolate reductase (MTHFR). Thrombosis and Haemostasis. 1997;**78**(1):523-526

[56] Pezzini A, Del Zotto E, Padovani A. Homocysteine and cerebral ischemia: Pathogenic and therapeutical implications. Current Medicinal Chemistry. 2007;**14**(3):249-263

[57] Suwelack B, Gerhardt U, Witta J, Rahn KH, Hohage H. Effect of homocysteine on carotid intima-media thickness after renal transplantation. Clinical Transplantation. 2000;**14**(6):555-560

[58] Schnyder G, Flammer Y, Roffi M, Pin R, Hess OM. Plasma homocysteine levels and late outcome after coronary angioplasty. Journal of the American College of Cardiology. 2002;**40**(10):1769-1776

[59] Selhub J. The many facets of hyperhomocysteinemia: Studies from the Framingham cohorts. The Journal of Nutrition. 2006;**136**(6):1726S-1730S

[60] Apeland T, Mansoor MA, Strandjord RE. Antiepileptic drugs as independent predictors of plasma total homocysteine levels. Epilepsy Research. 2001;**47**(1-2):27-35

[61] Basu TK, Makhani N, Sedgwick G. Niacin (nicotinic acid) in non-physiological doses causes hyperhomocysteineaemia in Sprague–Dawley rats. The British Journal of Nutrition. 2002;**87**(2):115-119

[62] Foucher C, Brugere L, Ansquer J-C. Fenofibrate, homocysteine and renal function. Current Vascular Pharmacology. 2010;**8**(5):589-603

[63] Müller T, Woitalla D, Fowler B, Kuhn W. 3-OMD and homocysteine plasma levels in parkinsonian patients. Journal of Neural Transmission. 2002;**109**(2):175-179

[64] Huang E-J, Kuo W-W, Chen Y-J, Chen T-H, Chang M-H, Lu M-C, et al. Homocysteine and other biochemical parameters in type 2 diabetes mellitus with different diabetic duration or diabetic retinopathy. Clinica Chimica Acta. 2006;**366**(1-2):293-298

[65] Masuda Y, Kubo A, Kokaze A, Yoshida M, Fukuhara N, Takashima Y. Factors associated with serum total homocysteine level in type 2 diabetes. Environmental Health and Preventive Medicine. 2008;**13**(3):148

[66] Niittynen L, Nurminen M-L, Korpela R, Vapaatalo H. Role of arginine, taurine 4 and homocysteine in cardiovascular diseases. Annals of Medicine. 1999;**31**(5):318-326

[67] D'agostino RB, Wolf PA, Belanger AJ, Kannel WB. Stroke risk profile: Adjustment for antihypertensive medication. The Framingham study. Stroke. 1994;**25**(1):40-43

[68] Wolf PA, D'Agostino RB, Belanger AJ, Kannel WB. Probability of stroke: A risk profile from the Framingham study. Stroke. 1991;**22**(3):312-318

[69] Fine-Edelstein J, Wolf P, O'leary D, Poehlman H, Belanger A, Kase C, et al. Precursors of extracranial carotid atherosclerosis in the Framingham study. Neurology. 1994;**44**(6):1046-1050

[70] Zhu Z-Q, Chen L-S, Wang H, Liu F-M, Luan Y, Wu L-L, et al. Carotid stiffness and atherosclerotic risk: Non-invasive quantification with ultrafast ultrasound pulse wave velocity. European Radiology. 2018;**29**(3):1507-1517

[71] Landmesser U, Hornig B, Drexler H. Endothelial function: A critical determinant in atherosclerosis? Circulation. 2004;**109**(21 suppl 1):27-33

[72] Elsharawy MA, Alkhadra AH, Ibrahim MFA, Selim F, Hassan K, Elsaid AS, et al. Impact of atherosclerosis risk factors on the clinical presentation of arterial occlusive disease in Arabic patients. The International Journal of Angiology: Official Publication of the International College of Angiology, Inc. 2008;**17**(4):203

[73] Słomka T, Drelich-Zbroja A, Jarząbek M, Szczerbo-Trojanowska M. Intima–media complex thickness and carotid atherosclerotic plaque formation in Lublin's population in the context of selected comorbidities. Journal of Ultrasonography. 2018;**18**(73):133-139

[74] Walker MD, Marler JR, Goldstein M, Grady PA, Toole JF, Baker WH, et al. Endarterectomy for asymptomatic carotid artery stenosis. Journal of the American Medical Association. 1995;**273**(18):1421-1428

[75] Collaborators NASCET. Beneficial effect of carotid endarterectomy in symptomatic patients with high-grade carotid stenosis. The New England Journal of Medicine. 1991;**325**(7):445-453

[76] Turtzo LC, McCullough LD. Sex differences in stroke. Cerebrovascular Diseases. 2008;**26**(5):462-474

[77] Hellings WE, Pasterkamp G, Verhoeven BA, De Kleijn DP, De Vries J-PP, Seldenrijk KA, et al. Gender-associated differences in plaque phenotype of patients undergoing carotid endarterectomy. Journal of Vascular Surgery. 2007;**45**(2):289-296

[78] Wild RA, Reis SE. Estrogens, progestins, selective estrogen receptor modulators, and the arterial tree. American Journal of Obstetrics and Gynecology. 2001;**184**(5):1031-1039

[79] Pines A, Bornstein NM, Shapira I. Menopause and ischaemic stroke: Basic, clinical and epidemiological considerations. The role of hormone replacement. Human Reproduction Update. 2002;**8**(2):161-168

[80] Anand SS, Yusuf S, Vuksan V, Devanesen S, Teo KK, Montague PA, et al. Differences in risk factors, atherosclerosis, and cardiovascular disease between ethnic groups in Canada: The study of health assessment and risk in ethnic groups (SHARE). The Lancet. 2000;**356**(9226):279-284

[81] Kim SJ, Song P, Park JH, Lee YT, Kim WS, Park YG, et al. Biomarkers of asymptomatic carotid stenosis in patients undergoing coronary artery bypass grafting. Stroke. 2011;**42**(3):734-739

[82] Marcucci R, Sofi F, Fedi S, Lari B, Sestini I, Cellai A, et al. Thrombophilic risk factors in patients with severe carotid atherosclerosis. Journal of Thrombosis and Haemostasis. 2005;**3**(3):502-507

[83] Rahman A, Quraishi FA, Miah MNA, Hakim M, Saha UK, Akteruzzaman M, et al. Relationship between homocysteine and carotid artery stenosis in ischemic stroke. Bangladesh Journal of Neuroscience. 2012;**28**(1):1-9

[84] Wu W, Guan Y, Xu K, Fu X-J, Lei X-F, Lei L-J, et al. Plasma homocysteine levels predict the risk of acute cerebral infarction in patients with carotid artery lesions. Molecular Neurobiology. 2016;**53**(4):2510-2517

[85] Zhang J, Liu Y, Wang A, Wang D, Jiang R, Jia J, et al. Association between H-type hypertension and asymptomatic extracranial artery stenosis. Scientific Reports. 2018;**8**(1):1328

[86] Laxdal E, Eide G, Amundsen S, Dregelid E, Pedersen G, Jonung T, et al. Homocysteine levels, haemostatic risk factors and restenosis after carotid thrombendarterectomy. European Journal of Vascular and Endovascular Surgery. 2004;**28**(3):323-328

[87] Mousavi SA, Ghasemi M, Hoseini T. Association between plasma homocysteine concentrations and extracranial carotid stenosis. Annals of Saudi Medicine. 2006;**26**(2):120

[88] Selhub J, Jacques PF, Bostom AG, D'Agostino RB, Wilson PWF, Belanger AJ, et al. Association between plasma homocysteine concentrations and extracranial carotid-artery stenosis. The New England Journal of Medicine. 1995;**332**(5):286-291

[89] Samson RH, Yungst Z, Showalter DP. Homocysteine, a risk factor for carotid atherosclerosis, is not a risk factor for early recurrent carotid stenosis following carotid endarterectomy. Vascular

and Endovascular Surgery. 2004;**38**(4):345-348

[90] Jeong S-K, Seo J-Y, Cho YI. Homocysteine and internal carotid artery occlusion in ischemic stroke. Journal of Atherosclerosis and Thrombosis. 2010;**17**(9):963-969

[91] Mueller T, Furtmueller B, Aigelsdorfer J, Luft C, Poelz W, HaltmayerM.Totalserumhomocysteine-a predictor of extracranial carotid artery stenosis in male patients with symptomatic peripheral arterial disease. Vascular Medicine. 2001;**6**(3):163-167

[92] Aronow WS, Ahn C, Schoenfeld MR. Association between plasma homocysteine and extracranial carotid arterial disease in older persons. The American Journal of Cardiology. 1997;**79**(10):1432-1433

[93] Aronow WS, Ahn C. Association between plasma homocysteine and coronary artery disease in older persons. The American Journal of Cardiology. 1997;**80**:1216-1218

[94] Aronow WS, Ahn C. Association between plasma homocysteine and peripheral arterial disease in older persons. Coronary Artery Disease. 1998;**9**:49-50

[95] Aronow WS, Ahn C, Gutstein H. Increased plasma homocysteine is an independent predictor of new atherothrombotic infarction in older persons. The American Journal of Cardiology. 2000;**86**:585-586

[96] Aronow WS, Ahn C. Increased plasma homocysteine is an independent predictor of new coronary events in older persons. The American Journal of Cardiology. 2000;**86**:346-347

[97] Sasaki T, Watanabe M, Nagai Y, Hoshi T, Takasawa M, Nukata M, et al. Association of plasma homocysteine concentration with atherosclerotic carotid plaques and lacunar infarction. Stroke. 2002;**33**(6):1493-1496

[98] Bakoyiannis C, Karaolanis G, Moris D, Palla V, Skrapari I, Bastounis E, et al. Homocysteine as a risk factor of restenosis after carotid endarterectomy. International Angiology: A Journal of the International Union of Angiology. 2015;**34**(2):166-171

[99] Spence JD. Carotid plaque burden is associated with higher levels of total homocysteine. Stroke and Vascular Neurology. 2017;**2**(1):40

[100] Zhang Z, Fang X, Hua Y, Liu B, Ji X, Tang Z, et al. Combined effect of hyperhomocysteinemia and hypertension on the presence of early carotid artery atherosclerosis. Journal of Stroke and Cerebrovascular Diseases. 2016;**25**(5):1254-1262

[101] Alsulaimani S, Gardener H, Elkind MS, Cheung K, Sacco RL, Rundek T. Elevated homocysteine and carotid plaque area and densitometry in the northern Manhattan study. Stroke. 2013;**44**(2):457-461

[102] Yang X, Zhou Y, Liu C, Gao X, Wang A, Guo Y, et al. Homocysteine and carotid plaque stability: A cross-sectional study in Chinese adults. PLoS One. 2014;**9**(4):e94935

[103] Alvarez B, Yugueros X, Fernández E, Luccini F, Gené A, Matas M. Relationship between plasma homocysteine and the morphological and immunohistochemical study of carotid plaques in patients with carotid stenosis over 70%. Annals of Vascular Surgery. 2012;**26**(4):500-505

[104] Hayta E, Hizmetli S, Atalar MH, Cinar Z. Association of plasma homocysteine level and carotid intima-media thickness in rheumatoid arthritis patients receiving methotrexate.

Archives of Rheumatology. 2015;**30**(3):214-220

[105] Catena C, Colussi G, Url-Michitsch M, Nait F, Sechi LA. Subclinical carotid artery disease and plasma homocysteine levels in patients with hypertension. Journal of the American Society of Hypertension. 2015;**9**(3):167-175

[106] Memişoğullari R, Erdoğmuş B, Alp HH, Bilgin C, Arbak PM, Yavuz Ö. Serum homocysteine levels in highway toll collectors and the relationship with intima-media thickness of the carotid artery. Turkish Journal of Medical Sciences. 2008;**38**(2):133-137

[107] Yasemin K, Fahriye FÖ, Ali BK, Sema NA, Tuba Ö, Esra YD, et al. The effect of medical therapy on plasma homocysteine levels and carotid intima-media thickness in Parkinson's disease. Journal of Neurological Research and Therapy. 2016;**1**(3):10-19

[108] Mungun-Ulzii K, Erdenekhuu N, Altantsetseg P, Zulgerel D, Huang S-L. Asymptomatic Mongolian middle-aged women with high homocysteine blood level and atherosclerotic disease. Heart and Vessels. 2010;**25**(1):7-13

Chapter 11

The Role of Lifestyle in Development of Coronary Heart Disease

Sushama J. Bhosale

Abstract

This chapter focuses on the study designed to assess the role of lifestyle in the development of coronary heart disease (CHD). The data were analyzed to compare the patients of CHD with matched normal. Lifestyle is defined as the general behaviour pattern of an individual including health behaviour, job involvement and work style, social interactions, intimacy, locus of control and values. For this purpose the matching of patients was carried out on one to one basis and on the parameters of the age, education, family size and socioeconomic status. Total sample size was 162. To measure lifestyle, a structured interview schedule was prepared which included questions on the subparts, viz. health behaviour pattern, job involvement and work style, social interactions, intimacy, locus of control, values. The coding of the responses was quantified. The higher is the scores more is the risky lifestyle whereas lower scores indicate the healthy lifestyle. Qualitative and quantitative analysis were carried out.

Keywords: coronary heart disease, lifestyle, health behaviour pattern, job involvement, social interactions, intimacy, locus of control, values

1. Introduction

Cardiovascular disease is reported to be the leading cause of death in world. In 1998, 12.4 million people died of heart attack and stroke. Of these 78% were in low and middle income countries. The high income countries had lower death rates because of better preventive and treatment program [1]. Though, several clinical and biochemical risk factors have been identified, the role of psychological factors are also gaining importance during the past few decades. Several risk factors have been identified to be associated with coronary heart disease (CHD) which include causative risk factors (hypertension, hyperlipidemia and diabetes), conditional risk factors (triglycerides and lipoprotein), and predisposing risk factors (obesity, physical activity, sex, family history, socioeconomic factors, insulin resistance and psychological factors) [2]. Evidence of various studies has shown a strong association in psychological stress and CHD. Cardiovascular disorders pose a major health problem for industrialized societies in terms of excess of morbidity and mortality. It is evident from the review of literature that there is a strong relationship between coronary heart disease and some psychological factors. Psychological variables like stress, personality, anxiety and lifestyle are contributing along with high blood pressure, obesity; lack of exercise,

IntechOpen

cigarette smoking and high blood cholesterol to the development of CHD [3]. In present study, a comparative study is carried out between coronary heart disease patients and non-coronary individuals in relation to lifestyle.

Large number of clinical and biochemical factors have been identified in development of CHD, the role of psychosocial factors are also gaining importance during the past few decades. The World Health Organization has stated that since 1990, 80–90% of people dying from CHD had one or more risk factors associated with lifestyle [4]. Lifestyle is a way person lives. This includes patterns of individual's health behaviour, social interactions, attitudes, values, belief and essentially the way the person perceived by himself/herself and at times also how he/she perceived by others. Lifestyle is one of the major factors which have shown a strong association with CHD [5]. Lifestyle is based on subjective perception, is purposeful and goal directed. It is motivated by a desire to overcome feeling of inadequacy coupled with an urge to succeed. The general goals of lifestyle are to understand, predict, and control life and self. Lifestyle has been found, as pointed out earlier, to have influence on individual's health, adjustment to environment, psychosomatic and psychiatric illness [6]. Health psychologists found that healthy lifestyle and dietary intake are associated with positive effects on blood cholesterol [7]. Diet, sleeping pattern, smoking, and alcohol taking habits have a negative effect on health [7].

Russek and Zohman [8] observed in young coronary patients that prolonged emotional strain was associated with job responsibility. The Framingham study had demonstrated the significance of lifestyle, employment and interpersonal stress. By showing that in males under 65, aging worries and daily stress and tension were associated with a greater risk of developing CHD, while for males and females over 65; marital dissatisfaction or disagreements were risk factors for CHD [9]. A diet high in fat, obesity and lack of exercise increases the risk of heart disease. Tobacco use, whether it is smoking or chewing tobacco, increases risk of cardiovascular disease [10].

There is a positive relationship between heart disease and fat intake, obesity, smoking and lack of exercise. The relationship between smoking and risk for CHD is simple and direct. Smoking has several negative effects on cardiovascular system (MacDougall, 1983, cited in [6]). Job dissatisfaction and work load in males emerged as a factor of predictive of CHD [6].

In the present study, lifestyle is measured on the basis of heath and behaviour pattern, job involvement, social interactions, intimacy, locus of control and values.

2. Status in India

In India, in the past five decades, rates of coronary disease among urban populations have risen from 4 to 11% and four Indians die every minute due to heart disease. In India, 50% of heart patients are under 45 years of age [11]. CHD is emerging as a major cause of death in India. It has been projected that 15 years from now India would have highest CHD deaths compared to any other country [12]. ICMR and WHO have predicted that cardiovascular diseases would be the most important cause of mortality and morbidity in India by the year 2015 [13]. Data from Christian Medical College, Vellore and All India Institute of Medical Sciences, New Delhi, over a period of 30 years showed a decline in admission for rheumatic heart disease (RHD) and increase in admission for CHD [14]. A comparative study in Singapore on Indians and Chinese, revealed stronger cardiovascular reactivity to stress among Indians than compared to Chinese men [15]. Chronic anxiety and tension have been suggested as factors in the development of CHD. There is strong evidence supporting prognostic associations with social isolation and low perceived emotional support and unhealthy lifestyle behaviors in the development of CHD [16]. In India, it has been observed that there is age related increase in CHD. The incidence of myocardial infarction (MI) was more common in urban India than rural areas of India [17]. Studies in India have shown that heart attacks in India occur 10 years earlier than in West. Hence it is needed to undertake well designed prospective studies for evaluation of CHD in relation to psychological factors [18]. According to Theorell et al. [19], cases of CHD may increase from about 2.9 crore in 2000 to as many as 6.4 crore in 2015.The prevalence rates among younger adults (age group of 40 years and above) are also likely to increase. Prevalence rates among women will keep pace with those of men across all age groups. Data also suggest that prevalence rates of CHD in rural populations will remain lower than that of urban population [17].

In brief the rationale of the study is the limited research available in this area related to psychological factors in India. This study was carried on matched subjects to contribute to this significant domain of research.

Lifestyle is one of the major factors which have shown a strong association with CHD [5]. Lifestyle is based on subjective perception. The behaviour pattern of an individual as expressed by his motives, his manners of coping and other factors including values, social and family satisfaction, job satisfaction and work style are called lifestyle. In the present study lifestyle is measured on heath and behaviour pattern, job involvement, social interactions, intimacy, locus of control and values. Research work has been done linking lifestyle, personality and coronary heart disease. It shows that Type A behaviour pattern (TABP) promotes a lifestyle which facilitates exposure to range of social, personal and occupational stresses which emerges into a coronary heart disease. Wright's identified five separate paths to coronary artery disease that are inherited risk based on family history, risks that accrue from personal lifestyle choices such as overeating and lack of exercise, anger directed inward, anger directed outward that is combined with a sense of time urgency and chronic activation and the traditional Type A pattern identified by Rosenman and Friedman. Regular physical activity in the context of work, recreation or an exercise training programme is associated with a marked reduction in heart disease related deaths in patients. Exercise has positive effects on the cardiovascular system that reduce risk for coronary artery disease and myocardial ischemia. Exercise tends to reduce heart rate, it improves the efficiency of the heart and it reduces blood pressure. It improves efficiency in the respiratory system so that oxygenation of blood and supply of oxygen to heart is better. Exercise reduces weight and there is a beneficial effect on cholesterol, triglycerides and ratio of HDLs to LDLs. The National High Blood Pressure Education Program recommended four changes in lifestyle to help, prevent or manage hypertension, since hypertension is a major modifiable risk factor for CHD. These are weight control, reduced salt intake, increased exercise and moderate alcohol consumption. Diet has a direct and important role in heart disease that goes beyond cholesterol. A diet high in saturated fat increases the risk of heart disease and stroke. Gender linked risk cannot be changed but high blood pressure, elevated cholesterol and smoking can be significantly reduced by life changes. Simple adjustments to diet and exercise have positive effects on both cholesterol and blood pressure. Tobacco use, whether it is smoking or chewing tobacco, increases risk of cardiovascular disease. Passive smoking is also risk factor for CHD. The relationship between smoking and risk for CHD is simple and direct. Incidence of heart attacks and sudden cardiac deaths is directly related to the number of cigarettes smoked on a regular basis. Cigarette smoking is the most preventable cause of coronary heart disease. The Framingham data show that men who smoke have up to 10 times the likelihood of sudden death compared to nonsmoker. Smoking interferes with the oxygen carrying capacity of blood, it reduces bioelectrical control and finally smoking increases the tendency to platelet aggregation and clot formation. Clots increase the potential for thrombosis and fatal coronary. Russek and Zohman [8] observed emotional strain associated with job responsibility in young coronary patients. There is a positive association between job dissatisfaction and CHD. Karasek's group in Sweden [18] explored the relationship of the kinds of work stresses that may be associated with cardiac pathology. They had given a model which links high work demands with an inability to make decisions. Theorell's prospective study of 6500 middle aged males in Swedish construction industry found dissatisfaction with domestic and working life was predictive of suffering a myocardial infarction during subsequent 2 years. In a study of London transport bus drivers and conductors, results showed that bus drivers had significantly higher incidence of heart disease than bus conductors because of more responsible and stressful nature of their work. The Framingham study showed that men undergo in frequent work promotions sustained an increased chance of developing CHD. A supportive social network and having community ties promote emotional and physical wellbeing. Some studies validate positive relationship between social support and CHD mortality. Studies on marital status have repeatedly shown that the single widowed or divorced have higher CHD mortality rates compared to their counter parts. It was also found that interpersonal relationship and marital dissatisfaction or disagreements were risk factors for CHD.

The association between values and attitudes towards life was studied in cross cultural context in Japanese young men.

It was found that Japanese who maintain their traditional way of life, values and language after their emigration to US, do not have increased rate of CHD. In study of Japanese- American males found that those with the lowest level of social affiliation had double the risk of developing CHD. The rate of CHD mortality increases due to smoking, alcohol and foods rich in fats, less exercise, lack of control over one's working environment, reduced levels of social support, the cumulative life cycle experience of belonging to a social class or nation undergoing rapid urbanization and industrialization.

The main objective of this research was to study the role of lifestyle in development of CHD and hypothesis formulated was patients of coronary heart disease (CHD) would score higher on subscales of lifestyle as compared to matched non-CHD individuals.

This being a study on stress, anxiety, type A behaviour pattern and lifestyle variable of the patients of coronary heart disease (CHD) and their matched normal patients for the present study were selected from cardiac care unit (CCU) of hospitals from Pune city. During the survey for CHD patients 10:1 ratio of male to female was observed. As, there is a physiological cause that men having a greater risk of heart disease than women do, because, the higher levels of high density lipoprotein (HDL) cholesterol, which helps to slough off the more lethal low density lipoprotein (LDL), these higher HDL levels appear to be linked to premenopausal women's level of estrogen. Estrogen diminishes sympathetic nervous system arousal, which may add to protective effect against heart disease seen in women. So in the present study only male CHD patients were selected. Out of 121 male CHD patients admitted in CCU's of various hospitals in Pune, 81 CHD male patients agreed to participate in the present study. In the present study selection of 81 matched normal was done by keeping the patients in view. The patients and normals were matched, one to one on the variables of age, education, occupation, family type and socioeconomic status. These 81 male CHD patients met the inclusionary criteria, which were as follows:

Age: 30–60 years; education: minimum S.S.C. passed; occupation: employed; family type: nuclear family is staying with wife and children, and joint family is staying with wife, children and parent; socioeconomic status: minimum income

DOI: http://dx.doi.org/10.5772/intechopen.86866

Rs 10,000 per annum. The normals were selected after the medical checkup by the physicians who labeled them as normal as they were not suffering from any disease.

Following tools and measures we used for data collection.

Personal data sheet: A personal data sheet comprising 14 items was prepared and was required to be filled in by the patients and normal before the actual administration of psychological scales. The items were designed to get the information about age, education, occupation, family type and socioeconomic status.

Interview schedule: To measure lifestyle in CHD patients and normal individuals, structured interview schedule was prepared on the basis of operational definition of lifestyle. Interview schedule includes four subparts in which questions are formulated beforehand and asked in a set order in a specified manner. The description of interview schedule is given in Appendix A.

Description of the sub-dimensions is given below.

A. Health behaviour pattern: It includes information about sleeping habits, dietary habits, daily exercise, smoking habits. To find out health behaviour pattern three questions were framed to get detailed information about sleeping habits, four questions for dietary habit, four questions for daily exercise, six questions for smoking habits. The coding of the responses is quantified. A five point rating scale, that is, always, often, sometimes, rarely, and never is used to measure the responses of person. Higher the scores on sleeping habits, dietary habits and smoking habits indicates more risky lifestyle whereas lower scores indicate healthy lifestyle. Lower scores on daily exercise indicate healthy lifestyle where as higher scores indicate more risky lifestyle.

B. Social interactions: It includes the information about social awareness and social life of the person. To get detailed information about social interactions 16 questions were framed. The coding of the responses is quantified. A five point rating scale is used to measure the responses of the person. Higher scores on social interactions indicate healthy lifestyle whereas lower scores indicate more risky lifestyle.

C. Intimacy: It includes the information about family and personal life activities. Intimacy is that quality of being close and affectionate with another person. It can occur with or without sexuality. To get detailed information eight questions were framed. The coding of the responses is quantified. A five point rating scale is used to measure the responses of the person. Higher scores on intimacy indicate healthy lifestyle whereas lower scores indicates more risky lifestyle.

D. Locus of control: It includes information about the individuals own interpretation of personal control over illness and health. Locus of control refers to the belief about location of control of behaviour by the subject. This locus is classified as external and internal. Individuals with external control think that their behaviour is controlled by the external forces like chance, luck, fate, some influential person or external circumstances. Individuals with internal control believe that their behaviour is controlled by the forces which are within themselves and the event is contingent upon their own behaviour. Eleven questions were framed to get detailed information about locus of control related to health and illness aspects. A five point rating scale is used to measure the responses of the person. Higher scores indicate internal locus of control whereas lower scores indicate external locus of control.

E. Values: It includes the information of two values namely money and religion of the person. Values hold a central place in culture, identity and lifestyle of the individual. Total eight questions were framed to get details about values of person out of which four questions were framed to get details about money and remaining four questions were framed to get details about religious values. A five point rating scale is used to measure the responses of the person. Higher the scores on money and religious value more risky lifestyle whereas lower scores indicate healthy lifestyle. Split half reliability was calculated and it is 0.89.

3. Procedure

A special permission was sought to collect the data of CHD male patients from cardiac care unit (CCU) of Pune city which includes Ruby Hall Clinic, Jahangir Hospital, DinDayal Heart Institute, Dinanath Mangeshkar Hospital, Joshi Hospital, Kashibai Navale Hospital and Sasoon Hospital.

On the initial contact, after noting down residential address of the patients, a formal permission was sought to see them at home after discharge from CCU within 10 days. Special visits were made to see the CHD patients from Khadki, Dapodi, Aund, Pimpari, Chinchwad, Vishrantwadi and Katraj in Pune city to interview and complete the psychological measures. After establishing proper rapport and explaining the objectives and purpose of the study the patients of CHD co-operated whole heartedly. All the scales and interview schedule used for this study were given individually to each patient at his residence. All the patients were assured that information given by them would be kept confidential and utilized solely for research purpose only. They were also instructed to ask for clarification of any doubtful item, specific instructions for each scale were printed at the beginning of the scale. No time limit was imposed for the completion of the scales.

Immediately within a week the sample of Non-CHD individuals were selected after medical checkup by the physician who labeled them as normal as they were not suffering from any disease. The patients and Non-CHD individuals were matched one to one on each of the variables of age, education, occupation, family type and socioeconomic status. A matched normal was assessed by psychological tests and was interviewed personally by visiting their houses. Initially it was proposed to take 75 numbers of data for both CHD patients and matched normal. But effective rapport and co-operation by CHD patients and matched non-CHD individuals the sample size was increased to 85, out of which four were rejected because the questionnaires were incomplete. In the present study the no of CHD patients were 81 and matched Non-CHD individuals were 81. So the total sample size was 162.

3.1 Analysis of data

Data were analyzed with the help of statistical techniques like descriptive statistics, and 't' test. However, a few cases were explained to understand the qualitative analysis.

4. Qualitative analysis

Analysis of personal data sheet was carried out. A personal data sheet comprising 14 items was prepared. The information in the personal data sheet was sought in order to match patients of CHD and non-CHD individuals on age, education, type of family and socioeconomic status.

4.1 Demographic characteristics of the sample

Table 1 and **Figure 1** show age group wise sample distribution. Fifty percent respondents belonged to the age group of 40–50 years. Similarly 14.8% belonged to 30–40 years of age, and 34.6% belonged to 50–60 years of age.

Table 2 and **Figure 2** show that there are 53% participants who are having PG education. There are 35.8% participants who were having graduation and remaining 11.2% participants who had completed H.S.C or diploma.

Table 3 and **Figure 3** show that 71.6% participants belonged to the nuclear family. Similarly 28.4% belonged to joint family.

Table 4 and **Figure 4** show socioeconomic status wise sample distribution. 4.9% respondents belonged to the 1,00,000–3,00,000 annual income group. 38.4% respondents belonged to the 3,00,000–6,00,000 annual income group. 35.8% respondents belonged to the 6,00,000–9,00,000 annual income group and similarly 20.9% respondents belonged to 9,00,000 and above annual income group.

Two case studies have been given to understand experiences of CHD male patients in greater detail. As mentioned earlier, a lifestyle was referred as a general behaviour pattern of an individual which includes health behaviour pattern, job involvement and work style, social interactions, intimacy, locus of control and values. Health behaviour pattern is a set of habits includes sleeping habits, dietary habits, daily exercise, smoking habit and physical and mental health.

4.1.1 Case study 1

A CHD patient of 37 years old working as a senior manager from last 2 years. He represents a nuclear family having a wife and a daughter. He had no family history of any disease. He is non-vegetarian and most of the time had outside eatables. He is a chain smoker. He is workaholic, carrier and money oriented and no time to spend with his family. A matched non-CHD individual also non vegetarian but most of time take his meal with family and rarely had outside eatables. He does not have any bad habit like smoking, chewing tobacco, etc. He had perfect compartment of work place and for family. He spends his weekends with picnic, get-together with friends, His priority to people and money.

Age group (years)	CHD patients	Non-CHD individuals
30–40	12	12
40–50	41	41
50–60	28	28

Table 1.
Sample distribution according to age (N = 162).

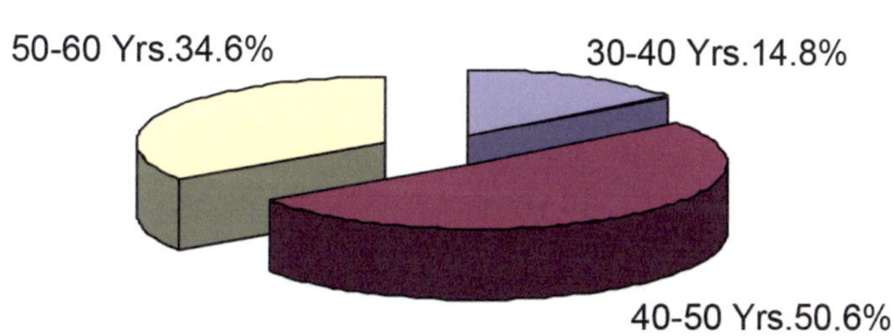

Figure 1.
Sample distribution according to age.

Education	CHD patients	Non-CHD individuals
H.S.C./Diploma	09	09
Graduation	43	43
Postgraduation	29	29

Table 2.
Sample distribution according to education (N = 162).

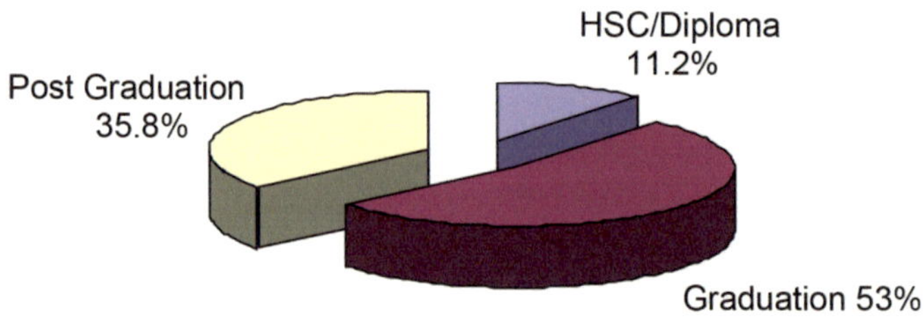

Figure 2.
Sample distribution according to education.

	CHD patients	Non-CHD individuals
Joint family	23	23
Nuclear family	58	58

Table 3.
Sample distribution according to family type (N = 162).

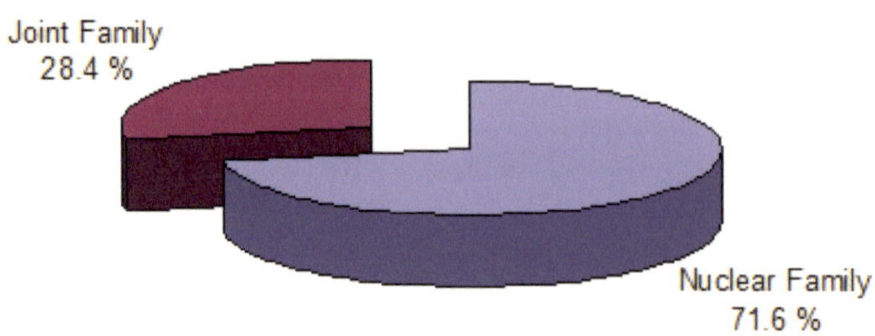

Figure 3.
Sample distribution according to family type.

4.1.2 Case study 2

A CHD patient of 45 years working as a senior lecturer from last 14 years. He represents a nuclear family of a wife and two daughters. He had no family history of any disease. He is vegetarian, not spend a single minute for exercise. He always chews tobacco. He is very competitive and always feels unhappy about his life and feels unlucky. He is religious and always depends on god. "I am very unlucky." "Asel debauch manat tar milel" such type of dialog often with him. He does not spend money, always worried about dowry and marriage of daughters. A matched Non-CHD individual is vegetarian as well as non-vegetarian. He daily takes a walk for half an hour. He is happy go lucky enjoy all the moments and takes responsibility of his work. The qualitative description of the two representative cases of CHD and non-CHD groups clearly demonstrates the noticeable differences in lifestyle factors. Results have been now discussed quantitatively.

Annual income	CHD patients	Non-CHD individuals
1,00,000–3,00,000	04	04
3,00,000–6,00,000	31	31
6,00,000–9,00,000	29	29
9,00,000 & above	17	17

Table 4.
Sample distribution according to socio-economic status (N = 162).

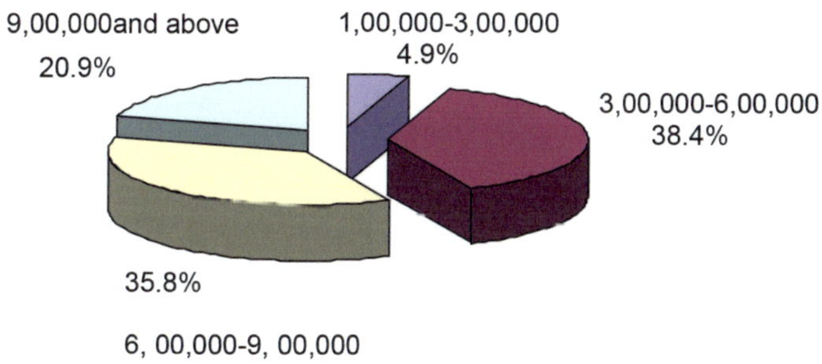

Figure 4.
Socio-economic status and percentage of people.

5. Quantitative analysis

5.1 Lifestyle among patients of CHD and matched non-CHD individuals

The results of present study indicate that the mean differences were statistically significant for subscales of lifestyle.

With reference to **Table 5**, CHD and lifestyle risk factors showed a significant positive association with sleeping habits, dietary habits, exercise and Smoking respectively. It was also appeared that there was a positive link between poor social interactions, poor intimacy, more external locus of control and more money and religious values. So, the hypothesis, "Patients of Coronary Heart Disease (CHD) would score higher on subscales of lifestyle as compared to matched Non-CHD individuals" is accepted.

The results of the present study support the findings of the earlier studies in association with lifestyle and risk of coronary heart disease (CHD). Gupta and Gupta [18] carried out a study on Indian male. In the present study, it was found that lifestyle risk factors like diet, smoking habits plays an important role in development of CHD. Orth-Gomer et al. [20] have demonstrated that low social support and poor social integration predicted incidence of major coronary events. The results revealed that the patients of CHD showed significant differences on locus of control, it indicates that the patients were titled towards external locus of control due to which they experienced the high stress on the other hand the matched non-CHD individuals due to their internal locus of control experienced less amount of stress and remain healthy [21]. The obtained results were discussed in the light of violation of assumption and compared with the results of earlier studies with necessary caution. A positive family history of premature coronary heart disease is recognized as an independent predictor for cardiovascular mortality in the first degree relatives. This will enable public health and behavioral epidemiologists to plan and target appropriate and effective preventive lifestyle

Lifestyle	CHD patients		Non-CHD individuals		t ratio
	Mean	SD	Mean	SD	
Sleeping habit	12.02	1.71	5.40	1.35	27.01**
Dietary habit	22.44	2.20	9.41	2.16	37.10**
Daily exercise	9.42	1.49	5.16	1.20	19.90**
Smoking habit	26.88	4.50	13.04	2.14	24.98**
Health	12.40	2.19	7.64	1.77	15.15**
Job style	65.30	10.53	33.90	5.66	23.61**
Social interactions	62.74	7.92	26.35	3.88	37.09**
Intimacy	21.75	2.92	12.31	2.17	23.32**
Locus of control	43.68	4.94	18.05	4.42	31.43**
Values	21.89	4.08	13.14	3.36	14.88**

**$P < 0.01$.

Table 5.
Means, SDs, and 't' ratios on lifestyle for CHD patients and matched non-CHD individuals.

techniques to adults. Therefore, its primary prevention is an important factor. Several studies have shown that primary prevention of coronary heart disease by family life education in the community has better benefits compared to secondary prevention for cardiovascular mortality as well as morbidity. Prevention programmers should have a multi-level focus, including individual, family and other social institutions. It is also important to identify subgroups for intervention, so that necessary steps at earlier level itself can be taken for the prevention of lifestyle diseases like coronary heart disease.

5.2 Limitations

CHD is a life time disorder; it is difficult to detect the sufferer as this illness does not reveal any overt causal symptoms. Moreover to get the authentic data, it was highly essential to consult the medical practitioners or cardiologists. Therefore, the researcher had to fully depend upon on the data which was available only in hospitals and clinics.

1. As mentioned in literature, the incidence of CHD is a global health problem which is given only medical attention, the psychological part of it is almost neglected. Though there are many psychological dimensions to it, only lifestyle has been studied in the present research, the other dimensions also needed to be studied.

2. The research is based on the data from Pune only.

3. This study was limited to male population only.

5.3 Implications

Healthy behaviour patterns like sufficient sleep, healthy diet, regular exercise, more social interactions, intimacy, and internal locus of control have beneficial effects among the non-CHD individuals. It is therefore reasonable to promote such a healthy lifestyle to the patients of CHD.

5.4 Suggestions

The following suggestions are made for future research:

1. Further research in this area may examine effects of emotions and coping behaviour in the development of coronary heart disease.

2. A comparison could make on urban and rural population to find out development of coronary heart disease.

3. A similar study may be conducted on a sample of female.

4. The further research in coronary heart disease may use multidimensional model encompassing both environmental variables (stressors) and social variables.

Appendix A

A.INTERVIEW SCHEDULE

A. Health Behaviour Pattern

i. Sleeping Habits

1. Daily hrs. of sleep: Sleeping Time: Getting Time:

2. Are you sleeping well? Yes/No.

   Always/Often/Sometimes/Rarely/Never

   If No, Why?

3. Do you sleep at daytime? Yes/No

   Always/Often/Sometimes/Rarely/Never

ii. Dietary Habits

1. Are you veg/non veg/mixed?

   If nonveg, How many times in a week?

2. Are you eating well? Yes/No

   Always/Often/Sometimes/Rarely/Never

   If No, Why?

3. Do you take your meal alone/with family/with friends? Yes/No

   Always/Often/Sometimes/Rarely/Never

4. Do you have outside eatables? Yes/No

   Always/Often/Sometimes/Rarely/Never

iii. Daily Exercise

1. Are you doing daily exercise? Yes/No

   Always/Often/Sometimes/Rarely/Never

2. Lonely/With friends?

3. Daily how much time you spend on exercise?

   More than one hour/Less than one hour

4. Which type of exercise you do?

iv. Smoking Habits

1. Do you smoke? Yes/No

   Always/Often/Sometimes/Rarely/Never

2. How many times in a day?

3. How many times in night?

4. Is their compulsive smoking?

5. Do you chew tobacco? Yes/No

6. How many times in a day?

v. Health

1. Does your family have a history of illness?

2. Before this illness are you taking care of your health? Yes/No

3. Before this illness have you suffered from any minor/major illness? Yes/No

   If Yes, When?

   Which drugs you had?

   Intensity of illness:

4. From when, you are suffering from this illness?

5. Does your illness interfere with your life a great deal? Yes/No

   Always/Often/Sometimes/Rarely/Never

B. JOB INVOLVEMENT AND WORK STYLE

1. Is your present job as per your ability? Yes/No

DOI: http://dx.doi.org/10.5772/intechopen.86866

If No, Why?

2. Is your present job as per your experience?Yes/No

   If No, Why?

3. Do you have most risky work?

   Always/Often/Sometimes/Rarely/Never

4. Are you doing extra work than your seniors?

   Always/Often/Sometimes/Rarely/Never

5. Is your work challenging?

   Always/Often/Sometimes/Rarely/Never

6. Are you happy with your promotion?

   Very much/Quite much/Not much/Very little/Never

7. At what extent are working conditions in your organization?

   Satisfactory/Unsatisfactory/Can't Say.

8. Is there high team spirit in your work group?

   Yes/No/Can't Say.

9. Generally my speed of work compared to others is fast.

   Strongly Disagree/Disagree/Undecided/Agree/Strongly Agree

10. I experienced inability to perform my job.

    Strongly Disagree/Disagree/Undecided/Agree/Strongly Agree

11. I get support from subordinates for my work.

    Strongly Disagree/Disagree/Undecided/Agree/Strongly Agree

12. I get support from my seniors for my work.

    Strongly Disagree/Disagree/Undecided/Agree/Strongly Agree

13. I think my job is reasonably secure.

    Strongly Disagree/Disagree/Undecided/Agree/Strongly Agree

14. I do not feel burdened in my work.

    Strongly agree/Agree/Undecided/Disagree/StronglyDisagree

15. I plan my work in proper way.

    Always/Often/Sometimes/Rarely/Never

16. I do not depend on others for my own work.

    Always/Often/Sometimes/Rarely/Never

17. I involve myself in the work.

    Always/Often/Sometimes/Rarely/Never

18. Are you satisfied with welfare facilities (medical etc.) provided by the organization?

    Always/Often/Sometimes/Rarely/Never

19. If I get similar job in any other organization, I would like to quit this job.

    Strongly Disagree/Disagree/Undecided/Agree/Strongly Agree

20. It is difficult for me to seek balance between my family and career

    Always/Often/Sometimes/Rarely/Never

21. When were you promoted last time?

22. Have you liked promotion?

    Always/Often/Sometimes/Rarely/Never

C. SOCIAL INTERACTIONS

1. How many friends do you have?

   How many intimate friends?

2. Do you feel that your friends understand you?

   Always/Often/Sometimes/Rarely/Never

3. Your social interactions are----

   Very much/Quite much/Not much/Very little/Never

4. Is your wife supportive?

   Very much/Quite much/Not much/Very little/Never

5. I am happy with my wife.

   Strongly Agree/Agree/Undecided/Disagree/Strongly Disagree

6. I am happy with my family.

   Strongly Agree/Agree/Undecided/Disagree/Strongly Disagree

7. I have happiness about my job.

   Strongly Agree/Agree/Undecided/Disagree/Strongly Disagree

8. I have happiness about my physical health.

   Strongly Agree/Agree/Undecided/Disagree/Strongly Disagree

9. I have happiness about my mental health.

   Strongly Agree/Agree/Undecided/Disagree/Strongly Disagree

10. I have difficulty in managing my time.

    Always/Often/Sometimes/Rarely/Never

11. I spare time for my hobbies.

    Always/Often/Sometimes/Rarely/Never

12. Do you feel angry with some people? Yes/No

    If yes, Why?

13. Do you feel awkward with some people? Yes/No

    If yes, Why?

14. Social co-operation helps me in getting success.

    Always/Often/Sometimes/Rarely/Never

15. Do you more irritable towards other people? Yes/No

    Never/Rarely/Sometimes/Often/Always

16. Do you lose your patience with other people? Yes/No

    Never/Rarely/Sometimes/Often/Always

D. INITAMACY

1. Do you and your partner have friends in common?

   None/Few/Many

2. Do you think that you understand your partner?

   Yes, always/Sometimes/Rarely/Never

3. Do you feel that your partner understands you?

   Yes, always/Sometimes/Rarely/Never

4. Do you visit friends and relatives together?

   Always/Occasionally/Rarely/Never

5. Do you engage in outside hobbies and interests together?

   Always/Occasionally/Rarely/Never

6. Do you share with your partner the responsibility of looking after your child/children?

   Always/Occasionally/Rarely/Never

7. Do you confide in your partner about your personal problems?

   Always/Occasionally/Rarely/Never

8. Do you feel that your partner depends on you rather than her relatives for advice about family matters. Yes/No.

   If yes, Always/Occasionally/Rarely/Never

E. LOCUS OF CONTROL

1. Illness is a matter of bad luck.

   Strongly Agree/Agree/Undecided/Disagree/Strongly Disagree

2. If it is in your fate, you cannot avoid sickness.

   Strongly Agree/Agree/Undecided/Disagree/Strongly Disagree

3. Keeping good health is a matter of good luck.

   Strongly Agree/Agree/Undecided/Disagree/Strongly Disagree

4. I think I can control my illness.

   Strongly Agree/Agree/Undecided/Disagree/Strongly Disagree

5. I do not have detail information about my illness.

   Strongly Agree/Agree/Undecided/Disagree/Strongly Disagree

6. I think one can maintain good health by paying attention to nutrition, exercise etc.

   Strongly Agree/Agree/Undecided/Disagree/Strongly Disagree

7. God helps us to keep healthy.

Strongly Agree/Agree/Undecided/Disagree/Strongly Disagree

8. People can help each other in dealing with many diseases.

   Strongly Agree/Agree/Undecided/Disagree/Strongly Disagree

9. There is no use worrying about illness, it will get cured when the time comes.

   Strongly Agree/Agree/Undecided/Disagree/Strongly Disagree

10. I know the steps to get out of this illness.

    Strongly Agree/Agree/Undecided/Disagree/Strongly Disagree

11. Good doctors can cure most illness.

    Strongly Disagree/Disagree/Undecided/Agree/Strongly Agree

Whether you feel successful/unsuccessful in your life, give at least five reasons:

(F) VALUES

1. Give your priority to values given below.

   Money, People, Carrier, Religion.

2. Having a family is more important to me than having a carrier and money.

   Strongly Disagree/Disagree/Undecided/Agree/Strongly Agree

3. Money should be saved for old age.

   Agree/Disagree/Can't say

4. Earning money only through labour and honestly appears descent.

   Strongly Disagree/Disagree/Undecided/Agree/Strongly Agree

5. Participation in social ceremonies is useless. Yes/No

   If yes, Always/Occasionally/Rarely/Never

6. Man should behave according to religious beliefs?

   Strongly Agree/Agree/Undecided/Disagree/Strongly Disagree

7. To what extent are you religious?

   Very much Quite/Much Quite/Not much/Very little/Never

8. Keeping fast is necessary on main religious occasions.

   Strongly Agree/Agree/Undecided/Disagree/Strongly Disagree

Author details

Sushama J. Bhosale
Mamasaheb Mohol College, University of Pune, India

*Address all correspondence to: sushama952004@yahoo.co.in

IntechOpen

© 2019 The Author(s). Licensee IntechOpen. This chapter is distributed under the terms of the Creative Commons Attribution License (http://creativecommons.org/licenses/by/3.0), which permits unrestricted use, distribution, and reproduction in any medium, provided the original work is properly cited.

References

[1] Barker DJ, Cox V, Kumaran K, Osmond C. Fetal growth and coronary heart disease in South India. Lancet. 1996;**348**(9037):1254-1255

[2] Deepa R, Pradeep R, Mohan V. Role of psychological stress in cardiovascular disease. International Journal of Diabetes in Developing Countries. 2001;**21**:121-124

[3] Stephan J, David M, Christopher C. Stress and coronary heart disease. MJA. 2002;**178**(6):272-276

[4] WHO Reports. APA Press Release. Public Affairs Office; Pam Willnez, 2002. 336-5707

[5] Cohen J. The global burden of disease study: A useful projection of future global health. Journal of Public Health Medicine. 2000;**22**:518-525

[6] Rice PL. Health Psychology. India: Brooks/Cole Publishing Company; 1999

[7] Williams PT. Health effects resulting from diet and exercise versus those from body fat loss. Medicine and Science in Sports and Exercise. 2001;**33**:S611-S621

[8] Russek HI, Zohman BL. Relative significance of heredity, diet and occupational stress in coronary heart disease of young adults. American Journal of the Medical Sciences. 1958;**235**:266-275

[9] Taylor SE. Health Psychology. 4th ed. New York: McGraw-Hill; 1999

[10] The Vestfold Heart Care Study Group. Influence on lifestyle measures and five year coronary risk by a comprehensive lifestyle intervention programme in patients with coronary heart disease. European Journal of Cardiovascular Prevention and Rehabilitation. 2003;**10**(6):429-437

[11] World Health Organization. World Health Report: Reducing Risks, Promoting Healthy Life. Geneva: WHO; 2008

[12] Reddy KS, Yusuf S. Emerging epidemic of CVD in the developing countries. Circulation. 1998;**97**:596-601

[13] Dholapuria R, Raja S, Gupta CK, Chahar RB, Gupta R, Purohit VP. Atherosclerotic risk factors in adolescents. Indian Journal of Pediatrics. 2007;**74**:823

[14] Rissam HS, Kishore S, Trehan N. Coronary artery disease in young Indians-the missing link. Journal of Indian Academy of Clinical Medicine. 2001;**2**:128-132

[15] Bhishop GD, Robinson G. Anger harassment and cardiovascular reactivity among Chinese and Indian men in Singapore. Psychosomatic Medicine. 2000;**62**:684-692

[16] Scheiderman N, Michael H, Antoni Patrice G, Ironson G. Health Psychology: Psychosocial and biobehavioral aspects of chronic disease management. Annual Review of Psychology. 2001

[17] Ahmad N, Bhopal R. Is coronary heart disease rising in India? A systematic review based on ECG defined coronary heart disease. Heart. 2005;**91**:719-725

[18] Gupta R, Gupta VP. Meta-analysis of coronary heart disease prevalence in India. Indian Heart Journal. 1996;**48**:241-245

[19] Theorell T, Karasek RA, Baker D, Marxer F, Ahlbom A. Job decision latitude, job demands and cardiovascular disease: A prospective study of Swedish men.

American Journal of Public Health. 2005;**71**:694-705

[20] Orth-Gomer K, Rosengren A, Wilhelmsen L. Lack of social support and incidence of Coronary Heart Disease in middle aged Swedish men. 1993

[21] Younger JB. A theory of mastery. Advances in Nursing Science. 1991;**14**:76-89